SID GARZA-HILLMAN

Ultrarunning for Normal People

Life Lessons Learned On and Off the Trail

Dedication

In this book I refer to a race I direct, the Mendocino Coast 50K trail ultramarathon. Each year I watch incredibly courageous runners from all walks of life—seventeen- to seventy-year-olds—toe the line. These athletes continue to inspire, motivate, and instruct me in my own life, and they are a major reason I wrote this book. My hope is that more and more of us "regular folks" discover all that this sport has to offer.

Contents

Foreword

Every year Sid provides "life pacer" advice ranging from Small Stepping, changes in nutrition, and real-life solutions for ultra-problems. I am a walking example of someone who never thought he could finish an ultramarathon (any distance longer than a marathon). I am a straight-up procrastinator, back-of-the-packer, and last-picked athlete. However, I now know trail running changes lives. Nothing else compares to being in nature without a watch or phone, just you and your trail dog or a chatty cohort cruising down a single track, whether you're on the East Coast, the West (best) Coast, or anywhere in between or beyond. That feeling of simply enjoying nature with no care for pace or distance goes by many names all over the world, but where I'm from in Northern California, we call it "trail surfing."

Surfers, the ones with boards and wet suits, always talk about the rush of catching a wave, no matter how fleeting the feeling may be. But there's no such thing as a perfect day out on the water: just hours of floating and waiting for the next set, which never seems to come. Or countless attempts to paddle out into an unrelenting sea that seems to want you gone. Dozens of waves are skipped because another surfer had the better line. It's frustrating, tiring, and sometimes annoying. Sometimes you're cold, hungry, or exhausted (sound familiar to any runners?). Sometimes you go home feeling like you've accomplished nothing. But when you break through and feel that feeling, even for a moment, it's all worth it. It's the tiny moments, buried in an ocean of other stuff, that matter. And then, once you experience that feeling . . . you won't shut up about it.

Running is no different, no matter where you run or how far and fast you aspire to go. Every run, race, or, heck, even a single mile is filled with hundreds or thousands of tiny moments to throw in the towel. The essence of trail surfing—or any running, or just life, really—is just choosing not to quit. That's it. True trail surfing is working through the discomfort and finding that place where the downs feel easy, the flats feel easier, and the uphills are just a little walk break before the next cruise down.

No one represents the essence of trail running and ultra-races better than Sid and his crew in Mendocino!

Whether you run a few steps on the trail or one hundred miles up and down the peaks and valleys of a mountain range, you're a part of the club. Here at Healdsburg Running Company, we celebrate everyone who has the courage to take on a meaningful challenge. Every athlete who makes it to the starting line has undertaken something profound. From the front of the pack to dead fucking last (DFL), from the podium to golden hour (the final hour before the overall race cutoff time), every finisher has grappled with demons. Every runner has taken not hundreds but thousands of "Small Steps" on the way to the finish line. Without actively choosing to take each and every next step, you never will. Even the smallest effort weeks and weeks before race day can make a huge difference when the seemingly insurmountable task can be broken down into manageable pieces. Those small steps in training become giant strides in the face of a monumental challenge. I call this process "the law of the farm." You do the work, or no harvest.

This book makes anyone and everyone feel that, by taking small steps, they can accomplish anything, whether that is an ultramarathon or any other lofty goal in life. Thank you, Sid, for putting together a book that everyone should read, whether they're a runner or not, a book that sees the world through the lens of a lifetime, challenging people to become the best versions of themselves ... Even if becoming that "best" version involves sleeping in a van to wake up at 4:30 a.m. and run for a whole day while eating nothing but bananas, peanut butter and jelly sandwiches, or weirdly flavored sugar gels.

Take it easy, but Sid teaches us to just take it!
Trust me.

It's fun.

You're gonna love it, and average Joes and Janes can get an ultra done!

Skip Brand
Founder of Healdsburg Running Company
Director of Lake Sonoma Race Series

Introduction

When I set out to write this book, my initial idea for the concept was an ultrarunning guide for people without a death wish. Let's face it: most people perceive trail ultrarunners and ultrarunning—distances longer than 26.2 miles—as an unattainable feat and that one would have to be detached from reality to even try. Many view it as a sport for got-something-to-prove type A folks and gluttons for punishment. Upon closer examination, however, a different reality emerges.

Though the world of ultrarunning has its fair share of elite and hard-core athletes, if you look close enough, you'll also find surprisingly regular folks: moms, dads, grandmas, grandpas, young, old. People with full-time jobs who lead busy lives while managing to successfully cross finish lines all around the world, including at the race I direct. So rather than embark on a more standard running guide—and upon further and deeper reflection—I realized that I wanted this book, on a fundamental level, to introduce ultrarunning to those who when asked about the sport, would respond that ultrarunning has absolutely nothing to do with them or the lives they live, that they'd never consider trying it themselves.

My goal is to demystify ultrarunning for all those who think that the sport exists in a world that couldn't be further away from the one in which they live, to relate it to those whose knee-jerk reaction is that they could never relate to it. Perhaps this is because I, too, was one of those people. When I unintentionally stumbled upon ultrarunning, I never would have dreamed that it would become such a powerful force of learning and growth in my life. But, luckily, I found it at the right place and time in my life—albeit it quite late. I discovered not only that ultrarunning is a sport that most non-elite athletes can do but also that their lives can be changed for the better for it. In fact, I would argue that as a species, we are wired for ultrarunning—and in this book, you'll find out why. By focusing on a philosophy behind ultrarunning rather than writing a practical running guide, I was able to move beyond boots-on-the-ground information (e.g., best running shoes and energy gels) and distill the lessons I have learned from my time on trails. Each lesson is one I did not expect to learn but one that has inalterably changed my life for the better. This is a book about how ultrarunning taught me to see the world—and my own internal world—in a different light.

Yet for those who, perhaps after reading this book, choose to attempt running an ultra, this book can be a helpful tool—just not in the way that typical running guidebooks are. In the following pages, you will not find charts, steadfast rules, specific race-day nutrition prescriptions, or running-gear recommendations. You will find practical tips and recommendations presented within the context of the overall mindset and philosophy I lay out in the book. In the lessons I have shared with you, I hope that you will find a new world of possibility and real-world advice that will substantially increase your chances of success not only at an ultramarathon but in your life. In this book, I use ultrarunning as way to frame the struggle of living a good, strong, healthy life in today's world by highlighting the intrinsic and extrinsic values of running on trails for long periods of time. Ultrarunning teaches us patience and perspective, the art of slowing down and paying attention, the power in coexisting with fear and in accepting the discomfort and struggle that are integral to a good life. Trail ultrarunning draws each of these and more out of every human being who attempts it.

It is true that trail ultrarunning exists in its own much smaller universe than road races and that most people are still not familiar with it. But our species is spending less and less time in nature, and we are the worse for it. Trails demand our attention, and the ultra-long distances we may run on them bring out of us a nature-based mindset that holds within it perspective, quiet, strength, peace, and focus—all of which are becoming scarcer with every passing day. The social nature of every race is real—humans crave and need to be around other humans—but even in the most heavily attended trail ultramarathons, we find ourselves alone and with only the sounds of nature, our footsteps, our breath, and our thoughts. Then, as the miles increase and the associated fatigue along with them, the average ultrarunner will inevitably be stripped of almost everything—will be laid bare, vulnerable, exhausted, and often on the verge of quitting. *Except*. Except there is a moment. A moment more physically and mentally taxing than most of us in our normal, everyday lives even get near. In that moment, most runners find a way out, or at the very least, they look for it. And it is that moment that answers the question of why we chose to try ultrarunning in the first place, and it is that moment that brings us back for more. It is that moment that inspired me to write this book.

The "we" in this book refers to normal people—hereafter "Normal People" because, frankly, we deserve the capital letters. If you were to look "Normal People" up in the dictionary, here's what I hope you'd find:

Normal person (noun phrase)

[nawr-muhl pur-suhn]

A person who has any of the following: a job, a family, or responsibilities and obligations that exist outside the world of trail ultrarunning.

We are the people living what may look to others like typical lives, but within them we hide a sacred, sideways glance in the direction of something else. Something more. We have jobs, some of us have children, and we have interests that lie well outside the world of ultrarunning. Most of us are not weekend warriors, type A go-getters, or adrenaline junkies. Yet something about a challenge lights us up. We have inside of us a deep-seated conviction that we are more than we think or even act like we are. Most days we may choose to turn away from this conviction or convince ourselves that it is not really who we are. But there is a fire within us. On paper it does not look this way. We go about the daily business of our lives, but in the background, we are thinkers. And when we successfully steal those rare but cherished moments of quiet solitude, we daydream.

I wrote this book because, for me, as for many Normal People, ultrarunning initially looked like a sport for crazy people, for the obsessed, for only those who are willing to put all their eggs in the ultrarunning basket. I wrote this book because of the countless funny looks I have received when people find out I am a trail ultrarunner. A great athlete, a natural athlete, a lifelong ultrarunner, they assume. No ... in fact, I'm a very mediocre athlete who found this sport at forty-five years old, squarely a back-of-the-pack athlete but one who has done the hard work needed to get to the finish line successfully. Oh, and I'm a father of three and husband with multiple jobs.

The world is full of incredible stories of elite athletes doing amazing things, but between these stories and us is a wide chasm. Their stories inspire us to be sure, but at the end of the day, they and we are not the same. However, while we are not elite athletes, there are very real, very meaningful elite parts of us, and we feel most alive when we strive to be the best versions of ourselves. As such, I believe ultrarunning is not only possible but profoundly beneficial for most Normal People. And as you will read, we do not have to drastically alter our lives to experience it. I believe ultrarunning delivers an awakening for Normal People that no other sport can, and the "why" will be revealed in the following pages.

Prologue

I wonder if I could . . .

As I stood at the start of the American River 50 Mile Endurance Run at six in the morning, one thought was front and center in my mind: this is the last place I want to be right now.

I'm not a morning person, and the 3:00 a.m. wake up, while not atypical for races—that is, if one gets any sleep at all—is never easy, much less pleasant. Not wanting to wake my wife, I got dressed in the dark hotel room, drank some water, and somehow managed to quietly assemble a decent cup of coffee. Coffee and I have a wonderful but codependent relationship: coffee gives me a wonderful taste and pick-me-up, and in turn I help coffee feel important. As such, I travel with my own coffee setup, an AeroPress travel coffee maker and home-roasted and freshly ground coffee. I refuse to subject myself to a cup of hotel "coffee," especially at 3:00 a.m. But even with my own setup, the coffee wasn't sitting well with my queasy stomach and only added to my bad mood, which I didn't shake until well into the race.

I hauled myself onto the school bus for the cold, long ride, then waited agonizingly long in a heater-less tent for the race to start. Prerace sleep is rarely sufficient, so I wasn't surprised to be tired. But, coupled with my ruffled mood and unruly stomach, the fatigue was palpable. With no chairs in sight, all I could do was lie down on the cold asphalt beneath my feet and wait for the race to start. As I lay there, I kept thinking of my wife in the comfort and warmth of the hotel room.

The gun went off for the first wave of runners, jolting me from my stupor. As a Normal Person, I was placed squarely in the second, slower wave of runners. The start of most races is a mix of nerves, anxiety, and excitement swirling around in a flow of adrenaline. I felt all of these, but another feeling was present, a weight against the buoyancy of the moment: dread.

Stepping over the starting line in a crowd of runners, I was so conscious—too conscious, perhaps—of what lay ahead. Fifty miles. Fifty. Miles. At the point I toed the starting line, the longest I had ever run was a 50K, about thirty-one miles, a training race I had completed about a month prior. Here, I would face *nineteen more miles* than I had ever run in my life. The pressure of this realization wreaked havoc on my mind and was only made more dramatic and dreadful given the exhausted state of my mind and body.

Still, off I went into fifty miles of hills, roots, rocks, and holes. Off I went into a sea of other runners that would soon narrow into a lonely, quiet solitude. The natural beauty surrounding me would not even enter my focus for miles to come. I noticed that many of the runners had arrived in groups and were chatting with one another. I had arrived, and I would finish, on my own. This was but one of the many times in my life I've felt alone in a crowd, and while I have come to appreciate the feeling from time to time, that morning's loneliness was amplified in a way that made me long for a running partner or group of friends to share the misery.

I reached the aid station at mile five and felt downright nauseous. I took a short break and decided then and there that the only way I'd possibly finish this race would be to focus only on getting to the next aid station. By mile thirteen, I began to feel slightly better. I hit a rhythm, and the chatter in my mind began to turn down to a manageable volume. As the sun rose, I felt my body finally waking up with it. But by mile twenty, the nausea and fatigue were replaced by a more general malaise—a physical manifestation of wanting to be anywhere else but running this race.

My wife joined me for a visit at mile twenty-nine and again at mile forty. Looking forward to seeing her kept me motivated enough to stay in the race. She shot some footage for a YouTube video I posted a few weeks later, and when I watched myself in the video, it was as if I were watching an entirely different person. Entering the aid station area, I looked downright destroyed but had a smile that seemed to say "What I am doing right now is insane." So crazy, so outside of my wheelhouse, so ... so ... I have only a slight memory of the actual thoughts whirling around in my brain, but watching the footage, I can tell that I was over it.

I remember striking a deal with myself early in the race—around the thirteen-mile mark, when I was in the throes of nausea—and it was this: if I encounter even the slightest physical issue, a hurt knee or twisted ankle, I'm out. I was looking for an excuse to quit. I was looking for a way out that would preserve my dignity, for a reason that anyone who knew I was attempting the race would accept without question. "Totally get it," they'd say. "If you hadn't gotten injured, I bet you would've finished, no problem." And somewhere in my brain was this conflicted desire for something, anything, to go wrong. Just give me a little pulled muscle, a twisted ankle, even a badly stubbed toe. I didn't want to actually get injured, of course, but I would have been totally fine with the prospect. Anything that would give me license to drop out without regret.

Instead, my training had paid off, which pissed me off. Aside from a couple blisters and a slightly banged-up big toe, the nail on which came off a few days later, I crossed the finish line without a twinge.

Crossing that finish line was definitely something. I cared nothing of the amount of time it had taken me, other than a mild appreciation for the fact that I'd been out there for eleven hours and fifty-two minutes. What I do remember and cherish was running the last twenty yards accompanied by my then eleven-year-old daughter. I heard my name announced over the PA system, and as I crossed the line, I was flooded with relief, gratitude, accomplishment, and a well-earned fatigue—a level of fatigue I had never before experienced.

The year before, when I was forty-five, I ran the first of only two road marathons I've ever run. Up until those races, I had run a few 10Ks and a couple half-marathons, but all few and far between. The common denominator in all those races was how I'd felt about them: I'd gotten very little enjoyment and experienced no emotional connection. I never finished those races and thought, "That was awesome! Can't wait to sign up for another!" I hated the pressure, the training plans, and the assumption that I needed to pay close attention to my pace during training. I viewed the shorter races merely as challenges I figured I should try, since running, albeit very recreationally, was a part of my life. It seemed to make sense.

The idea to attempt a marathon was the first of two running-related I-wonder-if-I-could? moments and was largely born out of dietary improvements I had been making. Previously marathons had existed only at the very edge of my radar—something I might do eventually. But as my diet improved, so did the speed at which I was able to recover between workouts. The stiffness and joint discomfort I had felt for years also decreased nearly into absence. With this new physical health and strength in my pocket, I seriously considered signing up for a marathon for the first time.

After searching for semi-local races, I came across the California International Marathon (CIM) in Sacramento. From what I'd read, it seemed like a great first marathon—an easily navigable "fast" course, not super hilly, not too far away, and recommended by some as a good first marathon. I looked into various training plans, settled on one that looked good enough to me, and followed it to the letter for about six months. In December of 2013, I jumped in the car with my family and headed out to Sacramento. That year was unexpectedly and atypically cold. Rather than warming to the usual forties or fifties, the temperature never exceeded low thirties throughout the entire race. Having not checked the day's weather report, I shed my sweatpants and sweatshirt at the start, and off I went. Unfortunately, neither Sacramento nor I warmed up that day. I remember having to ask an aid station volunteer to unscrew my water bottle lid for a refill because my fingers were too numb for me to do it myself. Farther along, the ground at each aid station had morphed into slippery layers of ice from the spilled water and sports drinks. It felt surreal to be sliding on ice through an aid station in Sacramento of all places.

In any case, I plodded along.

My goal was to break four hours, and while I came fairly close at four hours and eight minutes, my calves had begun to cramp severely around mile twenty-three, forcing me to finish the last few miles in a rotation of running, stretching, and walking that turned my frustration into disappointment well before reaching the finish line. I had followed the training plan and was confident I could do the distance. When I did cross the finish line, I returned to the hotel as quickly as I could to sit in a hot bath for over an hour, desperately trying to warm up. Despite the discomfort I'd endured, the experience seemed good enough, and I chalked up the cramps to it having been my first full marathon.

Not too long after CIM, I registered for my next marathon, the Avenue of the Giants, and in May 2014, I headed up north with the same goal of breaking four hours. This race was more my style: a gorgeous route through a thick forest of gargantuan redwoods. The course was entirely on paved roads, so while not a trail experience, running through a natural setting was more enjoyable than my first marathon. Spectators lined the race and cheered us on. I felt great starting out and fell into conversation with another runner for the first six miles. Unfortunately, this distracted me from my pacing, and I went out too fast—a common mistake for novice road and trail runners alike. At about mile twenty-three, I was plagued yet again with calf cramping and finished the last few miles in the same fashion of limping along as I had at CIM.

I'd accomplished two road marathons in the same year. I had answered the first of my I-wonder-if-I-could? questions. I could, and I did. However, I knew that I possessed not a shred of inspiration to do another; I'd closed a chapter. But a second I-wonder-if-I-could? question brimmed on the horizon, just out of grasp.

Soon, I would stumble upon trail ultrarunning: a sport, a challenge, a lifestyle that would change me forever.

Burned out on the grind of Los Angeles, my wife and I decided to move to a small rural town on the Mendocino coast. We had been in Los Angeles for twenty years, many of which had been incredibly fulfilling. My wife and I met while students at UCLA, and we both graduated in the early nineties. From there, we forged a great life. I pursued a music career while working with several other artists, actors, musicians, and general misfits at UCLA's Audio Visual Services until I fell into an acting career that surprisingly kept me working steadily for the next ten years while I continued with songwriting and performing.

We lived in Mid City, central to everything. We had a great group of friends, we loved going out, and we had an awesome little house with two detached garages—one a rehearsal studio for my band, and the other my wife's graphic design and letterpress printing studio. It was a compelling picture of a young, married, Gen X life. It was awesome, until . . .

Life in Los Angeles started to wear on us. The simplest things became a pain in the ass. A three-mile drive to the market regularly took over twenty minutes. A trip to the post office (just over a mile from our house) could take well over an hour. What had previously been just-during-rush-hour traffic became any-time-of-day traffic. Always driving around in circles in search of a parking spot sucked the energy from any outing. With the advent of reality TV, my acting career began to slow. And after the luxury of performing my music across the US, Canada, and Europe, I developed an acute distaste for the LA club scene, which more often favors commerce over art, and I stopped performing locally.

After a while, the nagging feeling that it was time to get out of Los Angeles grew in us both.

The nagging feeling came out of hiding during one of my very last acting auditions prior to our final departure, and I still remember it vividly. The audition was for FedEx, and I was going out for the part of a caveman. Unlike almost every other of the hundreds of auditions I had attended, where actors needed to show up looking only somewhat like the part, for this particular audition, we were directed to a wardrobe area where we had to get into a full-on caveman outfit. Picture Bamm-Bamm from *The Flintstones*—blond scraggly wig, leopard-print shorts, the works.

As I was putting on the wig, I heard a voice in my head exclaim so matter-of-factly that, after hearing it, I realized it was time to leave Los Angeles. The voice had said simply: "I'm so fucking out of here."

Soon after, we moved from the big city to a small rural town that, I'd soon discover, had a ton of incredible trails.

About four years before leaving Los Angeles, my wife and I had saved up for a trip to Scotland. We flew into London, boarded an overnight train to Edinburgh, taxied to the rental-car place, climbed into a compact Renault with a stick shift, and off we went. I could write an entirely separate book about my sleep-deprived foray into city traffic behind a vehicle with a right-handed steering wheel, shifting with my left hand. To make matters worse, we were confronted by our first superlarge roundabout. To call us "fish out of water" would have been an understatement, but once out of the city, we were taken by the natural, sparse beauty of Scotland. We found out-of-the-way inns and traversed a large swath of the country. We were smitten, but alas . . .

Back in Los Angeles, we tried for a spell to concoct a move to Scotland. We even picked "our" town: Ullapool in the Scottish Highlands, population of approximately fifteen hundred. Ullapool is the anti-Los Angeles but not so small that you'd know everyone within a month. It's a quaint town, somewhat populated, out of the way but not completely remote or cut off. At first, a move was a mere daydream, but soon we got pretty deep into logistics and practical considerations. Eventually, however, we faced a brutal truth: Scotland was not in the cards. We didn't have enough money to move that far away, and we'd have no prospects for work in a foreign country.

Still, we wanted to leave Los Angeles, so we considered more realistic locales to which we could feasibly relocate. My wife suggested Northern California, but for me (and many others from Southern California) that meant San Francisco, and I was having none of that. "No," she replied, "actual Northern California." I hadn't yet discovered the whole region of California north of San Francisco, some of the most beautiful country in the world. With the internet still somewhat in its infancy (dial-up, mind you), we began looking around ... for fun, or so my wife thought. I, on the other hand, was ready to go—especially after my epiphany at the FedEx commercial audition.

In the fall of 2005, three years after our Scottish trip and while I was on tour performing across Europe, my wife emailed me a link to a house she'd found in a little town on the Mendocino coast of California. It was so perfect I couldn't believe it: land, space, a big enough house, a basement with enough room for each of us to have a small studio, and financially possible.

Though my wife was still in that we're-just-looking-for-fun mindset, I became a bit obsessed with the idea that we could make the move. So, shortly after returning from my tour and after sufficiently bothering her by talking incessantly about the house and even secretly replacing her computer's screen saver with a picture of the house, she exhaustedly exclaimed, "Why don't you go up and look at the damn house?"

The following Monday, I flew up to San Francisco, rented a car, and drove almost four hours to the Mendocino coast, through some of the most beautiful country I'd ever seen. Wineries, redwoods, farmhouses, fields, and creeks gave way to rugged cliffs touching the edge of the Pacific Ocean. I had found, in my mind, Scotland in the United States.

Once there, I met with a Realtor, looked at and videotaped (yes, taped, as this was pre-iPhone) the "magic" house plus a few others, flew back down to Los Angeles the next day, and showed my wife the video. The video piqued her interest, and a mere two days later, we jumped on an airplane to visit the house together. By the time we returned to Los Angeles, we had put an offer on the house. The following day, our offer was accepted, and three days later, we put our tiny LA house on the market.

Six days after stepping foot on the Mendocino coast together for the first time, we had set a move in motion. It was that quick. It was that ill planned.

Up until moving to the Mendocino coast, I'd worked as an actor for ten years. In the beginning of my career, not having a "straight" job had felt very unsafe and totally unfamiliar. I never knew if or when my next paycheck would arrive, which was unsettling and not how I had ever planned to live my life. Like most people, I had figured that I would get a secure, safe job with a regular paycheck and try my hand at music, with low expectations. But acting quickly became steady enough that I was able to rely on it as my day job. For the next ten years, I was always a bit nervous about when I'd book my next job, and I even worried whether my current job would be my last.

Gradually, I came to appreciate this steady insecurity, and to this day, I still do. A heightened presence, awareness, and appreciation come with a little underlying fear, insecurity, and discomfort. I now see that there were distinct similarities between our sudden choice to move away from everything familiar and leaving my secure job at UCLA to make my living as a full-time actor. These two events—and, with them, my learning to become increasingly more comfortable with discomfort—inspired my foray into ultrarunning and the uncharted territory it represented.

A few months later, we were settled into our new house with our nineteen-month-old daughter. My wife continued with her design work, and I landed at the Stanford Inn & Resort, just outside the town of Mendocino. Knowing my interest in running and general health, Jeff Stanford, co-owner with his wife, Joan, handed me a *Men's Health* article about an indigenous tribe in Mexico who ran fifty miles a day—sometimes even running through the night—just for the fun of it. The article was written by Christopher McDougall who went on to write *Born to Run*, a book inspired by that same tribe.

The tribe, the Tarahumara or Rarámuri, lives in the Copper Canyon of northwest Mexico and is revered for its running prowess. Running is part of the tribe's culture and identity. It is cemented into its existence, both for enjoyment and utility. The Tarahumara will regularly run all day on trails, and in huaraches (basic sandals), no less. Even their very young children clock trail miles with relative effortlessness. Running intimately connects them to one another, their culture, and their environment.

I'm not sure what specifically drew me to their story, but the idea of running on trails was something I had not considered before. Trails were for hiking, or so I thought, and the fact that these humans were so naturally at ease running on them with no satellite watches, camel packs, extra-padded running shoes, sports drink powders and gels, nor all the other "necessities" intrigued me. I felt driven to experience even a fraction of what they might be experiencing. I wanted to find out if I, too, could run on trails; if I, too, could connect to nature in a way I had not yet been able to do, to feel a little more like a human animal and less like a modern human surrounded by comfort, noise, technology, and safety.

The article introduced me not only to trail running but also to trail ultramarathon races—races with climbs so steep that even pros will hike them. Races where people carry not only their own bottles of water and sports drinks, but also their gels, peanut butter and jelly sandwiches, bandages, extra socks and shirts, and more.

After the "meh" response I'd had to my two road marathons, and equipped with an improved diet and physical strength, I began to entertain the idea of trying one of these crazy races. Figuring it best to ease my way in, I began by checking out ultrarunning books and podcasts. The world of ultramarathons was fascinating right out of the chute. I was hooked. I soon became a regular listener of the *Ultrarunner Podcast* hosted by Eric Schranz. Schranz, who later became a great supporter of the race I created and direct (and who has even come out to run it), interviews all sorts of personalities in the ultrarunning world but especially professional ultrarunners. In fact, it was one of these interviews that inspired me to connect with pro-ultrarunner Matt Flaherty, who I ended up hiring for the first few months of training for my first race. Eric asked Matt about his successes and background and what was next for him, but the conversation eventually shifted to coaching. Matt explained that he coached both new and seasoned runners, and while he did help people with road races, his clients were mostly trail runners. Several aspects of Matt's story and coaching style drew me in.

He explained that he had been self-coached for the six years leading up to this particular interview—a six-year period that contained major ultramarathon successes. I was intrigued by this. How was it possible to be self-coached and still highly successful in this sport? Yes, Matt is an elite athlete, but the idea that someone could call their own shots in training was compelling to me. His approach resonated with me: he did not follow a one-size-fits-all strategy because, as he explained, everyone has different life stressors. Life stressors—not running styles, not baseline endurance markers, but life stressors like jobs and families. He was a coach who adjusted training based on multiple factors, especially factors that existed outside the sport of running.

I found in the world of trail running something oddly familiar to what I'd experienced as an indie rock musician. I listened to stories of so-called "professional" ultrarunners who lived out of their vans and traveled from race to race—the opposite of the slick, flashy, and polished vibe you might find in spaces where enterprise is the focus. I was drawn to what I perceived ultrarunning to be: an under-the-radar world, a subculture like indie rock. Neither world had become heavily corporatized, and both worlds were a labor of love and passion.

In ultrarunning, I found a community comprised of busting ass and testing your mettle, of dirty socks and bloody knees, and of tons of raw emotion. It was the anti–social media world. A back-to-nature and thinking world.

At least, that's how I saw it, and for the most part, I still do. I was drawn to it the same way I am drawn to my songwriting. There is a purity of solitude that is becoming more and more rare in other facets of life. Even now, in spite of an increasing presence of corporate sponsorship, ultrarunning is still *not* mainstream and still *is* full of singular characters and stories so compelling they read like fiction.

From the first moment of training, I felt like a fish out of water. Totally *not* an ultramarathoner by fitness level, athletic ability, or temperament, I was paralyzed by fear at times. Still, I persevered. For reasons I still haven't totally defined, I longed to be consumed by the soul of ultrarunning, because its soul is a conglomerate of misfits. It is punk rock music disguised as a sport, and a sport, I believe, that has hidden within it profound lessons. Lessons that, if we open ourselves to them, will positively and seamlessly improve our chances of succeeding in virtually every facet of our lives.

The lessons ultrarunning has taught me are many and life-altering. And each lesson came from one simple question that can deliver a long and fulfilling life to all who utter it: I wonder if I could.

To Move Through Fear

Fear is an extraordinary jewel, extraordinary something which has dominated human beings for forty thousand years and more. And if you can hold it and look at it, then one begins to see the ending of it.

—KRISHNAMURTI

Until one is committed, there is hesitancy, the chance to draw back, always ineffectiveness. Concerning all acts of initiative (and creation), there is one elementary truth, the ignorance of which kills countless ideas and splendid plans: that the moment one definitely commits oneself, then Providence moves too. . . . 'Whatever you can do, or dream you can do, begin it. Boldness has genius, power, and magic in it. Begin it now.'

— W.H. MURRAY

I was scared shitless, although, sure, first world scared. It is not as if paying a registration fee were some life-threatening

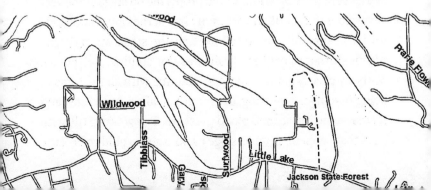

act. Yet the mere thought of committing to a fifty-mile trail ultramarathon—my first ultramarathon at that—was terrifying. I'd be going about my usual day-to-day commitments—family, work—and intermittent, random moments of dread would hit me. I felt the presence of a looming and gargantuan event in my near future, an event so outside my wheelhouse, it wasn't even in earshot.

How odd a species we are that we can exist in dread about something that we are choosing to do and that we are free to change our minds about at any time. Nobody was forcing me to run the race. Nobody was even daring me to. I chose it yet had to grapple with a future that was injecting moments of stomach-turning fear into my present. What I came to realize was that my fear of running the fifty-miler was so much more than the race itself. It was a fear that sucked into its fold ideas of failure, success, perfection, machismo, injury, embarrassment, disappointment, and even death. Fear that in an instant would drift into the paralyzing. All of this was set in motion the moment I registered for the race and continued until I crossed the finish line.

Why would I inflict this on myself?

The prefrontal cortex is to blame. Scientists call it the "executive function" part of our brain. I call it the part of my brain that, as a singer and songwriter, would propel me on stage at the very same time the reptilian part of my brain, the one responsible for basic survival, would tell me that the stage was a threat. Although that part of my brain was not "telling me" per se, my body clearly got the message, reacting with all the signs of being in danger: sweating, dry mouth, shallow breathing, and increased heart rate and blood pressure. The works. Still, with all of that happening, up on stage I would go. I would go because the executive-function part of my brain would "know" there was nothing truly life-threatening on that stage. I would choose to do something in direct opposition to what that bastard knot in my stomach was desperately trying to prevent me from doing.

The knot is a result of the lizard brain, the limbic cortex, the part of the brain that is there to help us survive when actual survival is on the line. Fight or flight. That part of our brain has protected our species throughout our existence, and in the wild, it does its job well. The hitch, however, is that in the lives of most Normal People in today's world, there is little by way of actual life-threatening stress, thankfully. No longer are we chased by predators, no longer are we in search of shelter, no longer are we in search of food. We have obliterated our survival-based stressors. How is it, then, that our species is more stressed than ever before and getting worse by the minute?

The epic, daily battle of *feeling* that survival instinct, that protective, instinct-driven fear—a fear designed to keep us safe and alive and somehow moving through this crazy world in spite of it, because we *know* better—is the very essence of the modern-world struggle. A lizard brain in a prefrontal-brain world. Our success as humans depends on an effective balance between the prefrontal cortex and the lizard brain. We must be aware of our fear while questioning it to determine whether it is valid and trustworthy. If we automatically give in to our fear, we never leave the safety of our rooms.

We win both individually and as a species when we learn to coexist with stress, fear, and discomfort in general. We better manage our stress (and therefore our lives) when we let go of trying to make all stress disappear and instead accept it and then learn to act in spite of it. A quote attributed to Eleanor Roosevelt reads, "Do one thing that scares you every day." To me, this means that we succeed in our lives when we refuse to be victims of stress and instead develop and evolve to become intentional, conscious, and active in our ability to live with it. It's as if to say "I'm not scared of being scared." I have learned through my own personal experience and while coaching clients that a significant portion of a Normal Person's stress comes from buildup we create in our own minds—the anxiety and stress we pile on ourselves just in the lead-up to what we think is going to be stressful. I identify this in my life as the intense fear I felt virtually every day as my first race approached that was independent of the fear I felt when I toed the line. When we learn to coexist with our fear and occasionally even *invite* it into our lives, we remind ourselves that we need not ever fully give ourselves over to it.

As part of the training for my fifty-miler, my coach recommended I run a 50K to gain some ultramarathon experience. A 50K is technically 31.07 miles, but rarely is any ultramarathon that precise. In fact, the 50K I direct comes in at around thirty-two to thirty-four miles depending on what GPS watch runners are wearing and how angry they are at me when they cross the finish line. I drove out to that race—the Way Too Cool 50K—by myself, spent the night in a crappy motel, and showed up to the starting line not having any idea how the day would go. How could I? The farthest I had ever run up to that point were the two road marathons, 26.2 miles each, and I'd never run anywhere near that long of a distance on trails. However, the fear was less intense because I considered it only a training run, just for the race experience and nothing more. The goal of the day was to get a sense for how these crazy things go, essentially a note-taking mission. I'd already put all my eggs in the basket of the finale: the American River fifty-miler that was lingering out there about two months in my future. Perception, perception, perception. A 50K wasn't so bad. It wasn't a fifty-miler at least, right? I marveled at how odd relative stress can be that a 50K wasn't very fear-inducing that morning.

Once I took off, I felt quite fine and ran the race smart. I followed my coach's advice of running the flats and downhills, then hiking the hills. The day was a success. I finished it well, and I'd barely glanced at the clock. It was quite liberating to be more than satisfied with the fact that I had not only finished but finished strong, with little concern for pacing. And while it was clearly not the "big" race for which I was ultimately training, a subtle switch went off in me as I crossed the finish line. At that moment, I became aware that even this race, this 50K training race, my first ultramarathon, was a bigger deal than I had anticipated. Crossing the finish line removed the *training* from *training race*, and the reality settled in that this was a momentous, out-of-the-box act for me. It felt really good and really profound. I felt a high that went beyond the endorphin rush runners often report about. It was a mixture of "Holy crap, what did I just do?" and "Holy crap, I just did this." It was at once a step along the way to my fifty-mile race and a self-contained accomplishment.

As I removed my shoes and socks—both with holes aplenty, as I'm one of those runners who wear their shoes until they are way past their prime—and climbed into my car, I realized I'd overlooked a detail planning my travel to and from the race. Rather than taking our automatic minivan, I'd chosen to drive the stick shift because it was smaller and more fuel efficient. Though a good decision on paper, the extra strain proved painful on my exhausted muscles. I yelped every time I had to push in the clutch pedal. The muscular fatigue was already palpable on the almost four-hour drive home, and I limped for a few days after. I'd learned that the reality of ultrarunning fatigue and soreness is that they are unequivocally earned. There is a next-level accomplishment attached to both, and their presence, while uncomfortable, was an oddly welcomed reminder of what I had just achieved.

Unfortunately, the feeling of accomplishment was rather short-lived upon my return. After a few recovery days, I eased back into training. Quickly, I was reminded that, while the 50K trail run was nothing to scoff at and a struggle to achieve, at the starting line of the American River fifty-miler, I would be facing a race with *nineteen* more miles than I had ever run before. *Nineteen more miles.*

Many Normal People might not know that runners typically never run the full race distance during training. Since most people train five or six days a week, attempting to run the full race distance on any given day would be a counterproductive push, forcing unnecessary strain on your body. However, the weekly mileage adds up to well over the race distance; in fact, weekly mileage for ultramarathon training floats around thirty to seventy miles. As a coach of Normal People, I am more concerned with overtraining than undertraining. Running most days *and* attempting superlong runs *and* working a full-time job *and* raising a family, and, and, and ... can quickly become too much. I admit there is a confidence boost in hitting the race distance during training, but for a Normal Person, I believe it's not worth the risk of injury or burnout.

So, there were the nineteen *additional* miles just hanging out there, slowly chipping away at whatever confidence I had garnered from my strong 50K-training-race finish. I still had no way of knowing if I would be able to finish the fifty-miler until, well, I either finished it or didn't. Such is trail ultrarunning ...

During my fifty-miler training, I was told several times that at some point during the race, I would want to quit. For real. I thought to myself, "Sure, but for real?" Would I truly want to quit, or would it be a general "This sucks. I feel like quitting, and I wish I weren't doing this, but of course I'm going to plug ahead" kind of thing? Turns out it was the former.

It is difficult for Normal People to wrap our brains around the idea that we will *actually* want to quit during an ultramarathon— not just count down the miles as fatigue becomes more and more palpable. Most of us will hit bottom at some point. A bottom we cannot even imagine until we are there, and one that most Normal People have never hit. One more time: most Normal People will *actually* want to quit at some point during an ultramarathon race (and, in fact, some do). And this is *not* a game. And this *is* something to fear. We fear the race itself, and we are afraid we may not finish. Like all unknowns, ultrarunning is too easy to perceive, on some level, as a threat to our survival. The relatively high level of comfort in our everyday lives keeps us quite far from any real bottom. The idea that we could be heading for one—by choice, no less—and that we are going to feel a low that is lower than we have ever experienced up to that point is a frightening prospect.

Normal People are afraid of this bottom, and rightfully so, because at this bottom we are subsumed by and consumed with inside pressure, outside pressure, fear, and intense discomfort. We are afraid of what it might feel like, and we're afraid that if we surrender to the feeling of quitting, we will feel shame, failure, guilt. And if we do not give in to it and instead forge ahead, we could open ourselves to physical injury. With each additional race, this whole picture becomes more perceptible and familiar, but it never gets much easier.

For any Normal Person even flirting with the idea of an ultramarathon, the question is likely "Why do it, then?" Here is why: if at the moment we feel like quitting, we instead continue in spite of it, then we see a power inside of us we never knew we had—and often for the first time. This experience is, I believe, the main driver of why Normal People continue running ultramarathons beyond our first attempts; we come to see a profound value in the periodic reminder of what we can accomplish and that we can indeed survive and even thrive in the face of adversity. We see that we do not have to let fear stop us in our tracks.

In my Small Steps coaching practice, I help Normal People become comfortable with discomfort. It sounds like a paradox, but the fact is that we have become not only more addicted to comfort but also unnaturally demanding of it. We have unprecedented access to highly effective tools that minimize or even erase even the slightest hint of discomfort—air conditioners, heaters, junk food, caffeine, alcohol, drugs, social media, and cell phones—all of which can have adverse effects on our health and happiness. When we stumble upon momentary discomfort, we don't look for the underlying cause. Instead, we look for a modern-world quick fix to rid ourselves of it immediately. Headaches, digestive upset, low energy, unfulfillment, and general unhappiness are no match for the technological "solutions" our species has created, and this is precisely why it is so easy to become addicted to them. It is just too easy to employ a drug that will obliterate the hard work of paying sufficient attention to how we live our lives and to the relationships, habits, and behaviors we engage in. Our species is largely able to "phone it in," and, as a result, we are becoming softer and less resilient by the minute.

Yet the underlying causes of discomfort can be the very knowledge that moves us forward in our lives. We should seek the information that, when addressed, helps us to live healthier, happier lives. Seeking this information means spending just a little time to ask why we aren't sleeping well; why we're drinking too much coffee and consuming too much alcohol; why we're constantly craving junk food and having headaches, stomachaches, digestive discomfort; and why we're feeling anxious, irritable, or restless. Seeking means bringing the potential causes of any of these to the surface so that we can confront and resolve them. Often, we need help solving these issues, and it is a position of strength to ask for help when we need it. If a Normal Person is striving for constant comfort, it usually means there is something lurking under the surface that is holding us back; however, we live our lives better when we call it out into the open.

My 50K experience was a success, but that very *low* low did indeed come. Just as I was warned it would, I landed in that dreaded moment where I truly wanted to quit, where the discomfort and fatigue were so intense that I truly did not know whether I had the strength to continue. I do not ever remember having felt anything even close to that, and I'd already lived forty-six years on this earth. The difficulty of the race fell far beyond my local trail-training runs. All of the factors—the unfamiliarity of the terrain; the fact it was simultaneously my first trail race *and* first ultramarathon; the mental and physical challenge of running farther than I'd ever run before; the substantial lack of sleep from the previous night, due to my prerace jitters; and, finally, the fact that I was doing it all solo, with no friends to run with, to travel with, nor to see at the finish—forced me to reach a low truly unlike anything I had ever felt before.

But the highs and lows that constitute trail ultramarathons are what make the sport incredible, what set it apart as not just an astounding physical challenge but an overwhelming mental game. During a race, you can truly feel like quitting one moment only to catch an influx of energy an hour later and feel like you are on top of the world. You can supposedly be on your last legs, barely able to walk, yet somehow run the last few miles, all because you know the finish is close. The lore (a "rule" Navy SEALs train by) is that when you feel completely spent, you are only at about 40 percent of your capacity. True or not, the fact is that when you think you can't continue, you usually are far from having reached your limits. It's a fascinating state to be embroiled in as it unfolds in real time, as if you were witnessing a play in which you are both the main character and the director. The play will most certainly contain action, fear, tension, tragedy, excitement, joy, and relief.

I finished the 50K in just under seven hours. During the race, the clock had carried no weight whatsoever except for the fact that I was a bit amazed to have been moving for seven hours straight. Crossing the finish line was as otherworldly as the fatigue, as was the profound relief I felt. Someone handed me a medal, and after walking a bit to avoid stiffening up, I phoned my coach to deliver a race report. By this time, we were no longer working together, but the training for this 50K had been set in motion on day one, and he, as an excellent coach, was invested in the process. The fifty-miler was looming, but the training thus far had paid off. In fact, precisely because of the training and the confidence that came with it, I had not been crippled by the fear that I'd felt when I heard the gun fire.

At the end of the day, all we have is training. How well we take care of ourselves, strengthen our bodies and minds, and nourish ourselves directly influence how we perform when we are thrust—by choice or otherwise—into any unknown. It is not just *sort of* about the training, it is all about the training. Just toeing the line that day was a big win for me. I did not know whether I would finish. I could not know. I knew only that I had trained well and that that was what had gotten me there. The rest was out of my hands. As the gun went off, I passed over the starting line squarely in a reality of not knowing. Though a scary place to be, I ran nevertheless because, with solid training under my belt, I felt that at least my *chance* of finishing was pretty good. A well-earned pretty-good chance.

In all of our lives, there is often something hanging around that, on some level, we would like to try but that we are terrified of trying at the same time. The trick is never to focus on making the fear go away, because in doing so, we waste so much time and energy attempting to *not* feel something rather than developing the strength to pursue the lives we want to live. In other words, the trick is to move through fear, to live our lives *in spite of* fear. Because if left unchecked, and with a ton of energy depleted in trying desperately to avoid or hide from it, fear will win the day. It will paralyze us. It will keep us stuck in our lives. We will not venture, we will not stretch, we will not feel. Kept in check, however, fear can motivate us to live more fully, more fulfilled, and happier. This in turn becomes a liberating and confidence-building habit—the habit of accepting the existence of fear in our lives and toughening our minds so we care much less about it over time.

For Normal People, there is so much unknown in ultrarunning. It is a sport that lives completely outside what we think is even possible. It sounds so incredibly crazy and like something that *other* people do. It lives completely outside of our everyday lives. For Normal People, an ultramarathon is scary. We can't even imagine doing it.

That is, until we do it.

Ultrarunning teaches Normal People to move through fear.of a particular race because not doing so would be risking too much. This is not only okay but it's the right thing to do. If you truly cannot go on, here is what you do: go back to the drawing board, retool your training, and try again.

To Slow Down

Slow and steady wins the race . . . Unless the race is, you know, being timed and other people are competing against you. In that case, speed is really more valuable.

—EXCERPT FROM A CONVERSATION BETWEEN ME AND MY GOOD FRIEND JIM ELDRIDGE … AND SINGLE MALT SCOTCH

Up until I was able to move through the fear and sign up for my first ultra, I had run only recreationally. I would run a few miles here, a few there. The scattered few races I had entered didn't take hold of me. I resented the formal training and running becoming a "have to." Whenever a race loomed in the future, I bore stress and pressure that never felt worth it. Sometimes the races were mildly fun, but they never left me feeling like I wanted more. Mostly I ran for exercise, for the physical benefit, and, as such, I thought of running as something to get done. But as a low-maintenance form of exercise, running is easy to find time to do, which kept me running often enough. All I needed was a pair of shoes, and I was good to go.

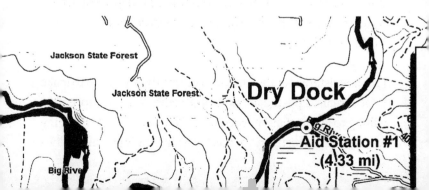

Running during college was easy—a run around the UCLA campus was safe, challenging, and convenient. Postcollege and beyond, I only had to step out my door on weekends. Several times over the years, I tried working out in gyms, but that never seemed to last more than a few months. The amount of time it took to drive to the gym, work out, then drive home quickly burned me out—and that was before I had children. Working out in the gym was prohibitive long term, so I always fell back on the logistical ease of running. My father was a road marathoner, so I had grown up around it. I remember going to his races and watching him finish, and one of my fondest memories is finishing a half-marathon with him as an adult. Running was familiar and made sense. Until I found trail ultrarunning, it was just the exercise I did, but it never carried anything meaningful or philosophical for me beyond fitness and health.

But with improvements to my diet, I began to feel pretty darn good—perhaps the best in my life—and I noticed how quickly and easily I recovered after runs. I was forty-four with no joint pain and more energy, and I felt less wrecked after long runs. With this strong foundation in place, I figured it was time to challenge myself and run my first marathon. Again, neither that race nor the subsequent marathon later that year hooked me. I never caught the marathon bug. But quickly after, I stumbled upon trail running, which could not have come at a better time. If I hadn't discovered trail running, I probably would have returned to recreational running and never experienced the world of trail ultras.

I soon registered for the American River fifty-miler, and to make it feel "real," I posted about it on Facebook. I was more than willing to admit that I needed help. The world of ultrarunning was uncharted territory for me, both physically and mentally. I was simultaneously taking on trail running and ultra-distances for the first time. I read some ultramarathon books, all of which contained training plans. I followed the plans so closely, so rigidly, that they became a detriment to my training and my quality of life in general. Quickly enough, when I saw the plan on the page, I began to detach from myself, from my own needs. The plan was the plan, regardless of how I felt or what was going on in my life.

Eventually, the sheer size of an ultramarathon coupled with my desire to break myself from the control of a chart in a book led me to hire a training coach.

By definition, an ultramarathon is any distance over the marathon's 26.2 miles. However, in the world of ultras, there tend to be fixed distances: fifty kilometers, fifty miles, one hundred kilometers, one hundred miles, and so on. (Why the switch between metric and imperial? Likely the purpose is to maintain clean, round numbers, as 31.07 miles does not sound as sexy as 50K.) And a trail ultra is, well, an ultramarathon that is run on ... wait for it ... trails.

A trail ultramarathon is a different animal than a road marathon. Not better, not worse, just different. I certainly prefer it for reasons we'll continue to explore. Because of the varied nature of trails, the training for a trail ultramarathon, in addition to banking more miles than one would during road-marathon training, involves developing multiple muscle groups. Consider the physical difference between running on artificially flat surfaces like roads, sidewalks, and treadmills compared to natural, uneven rock-, root-, and hole-filled trails, often with scattered severe hills and downhills. I had no idea how to train effectively or even where to start. But the power was in knowing what I didn't know.

Enter a running coach.

Matt Flaherty is not only a famously mustached ultrarunner but also a lawyer and musician. He embodies what drew me to the sport in the first place: a ragtag, living-out-of-a-van community of athletes. After hearing him interviewed on the *Ultrarunner Podcast*, I shot him a quick email about a month before my forty-sixth birthday, inquiring whether he had the space and inclination to take me on as a client. He gave me a thumbs-up, and we began training. It was an eye-opening, irreplaceable experience for me.

Up until the moment I began my training with Flaherty, my average pace was about eight minutes per mile—fairly speedy—and right out of the chute, he instructed me to slow down. I thought, "But I can go pretty far at an eight-minute mile, and I haven't even started training!" But he assured me that the approach had to be different because the race was different. This wasn't a few miles or even a few more miles. This was fifty miles. Fifty miles, all at once. I had not fully wrapped my inexperienced brain around the distance. My usual eight-minute-mile pace was doable for two to three miles, but could I keep that pace up for fifty? Not by a long shot. My usual pace was too fast to carry me into much greater distances with a similar ease. Even a ten-miler at that pace would be unsustainable. At least that much was clear.

So slow down I did, and significantly.

Soon, a new, unfamiliar goal emerged: to run a twelve-minute-mile pace. The first few runs at this slower pace were surprisingly challenging and, as one might expect, for reasons having absolutely nothing to do with physical strain. In fact, these runs were the most relaxing and low-stress runs I had ever experienced. My breathing was calm, my energy steady, my body efficient. Before tackling this new approach to training, I would finish a longer run and be tanked for a few hours afterward, but following these long, slow days (LSDs, as Flaherty called them), I would feel almost as if I hadn't even run that day. No soreness, no stiffness, no fatigue. At most, I'd experience only a minor feeling of being tired, which after a fifteen-mile trail run was mind-blowing.

As a Normal Person, I did not want the training to cut significantly into my family life. I was willing to sacrifice a little since this type of training wasn't a lifelong commitment; I knew that the day after the race I would return to my normal schedule of family, work, light exercise, and my usual free-time activities. The really long, slow run days were primarily on weekends, some of which were back-to-back long runs, such as running a twelve-miler on Saturday, then a fourteen-miler on Sunday. I made sure to leave early enough so that I would be finished around the time my family would wake up. The slower pacing was a blessing for my time with my family as well: I would return from these runs with plenty of energy for my kids and to run errands. Suddenly, a super slow fourteen-miler became no big deal. The fact that it was over a half-marathon but just one of my weekend runs did not even occur to me. In fact, I remember looking at a run Flaherty had planned for me the day after I'd run a fourteen-miler and thought, "Oh, thank goodness, I'm doing only a twelve tomorrow." This was such an odd reality for me to wrap my head around: that I was empowered to clock more miles with less fatigue and more energy.

But slowing down was challenging. Learning how to pace myself was a physical effort in addition to a mental one. I relegated my Suunto GPS watch, replete with a plethora of tools, data, measurements, and connectivity, to one purpose only: to remind me to slow down. During the initial slow runs, I would check the watch frequently to often discover that my pace had crept up, my body and muscle memory reverting to their routine and familiar pace. But slow down again I would. As with most things we stick with for a while, I eventually adapted, so much so that I no longer need to wear a watch, but this took time and concentration.

Learning to slow down was also a mental challenge. At first, I noticed a deep-seated machismo rearing its head—an intense urge to let everyone I saw on a run know that I could run faster if I wanted to. But the most challenging aspect was the silence. During pretraining runs, my pace was always fast enough to keep me distracted by my discomfort and the desire to get the run over with. But slowing down reduced my stress and discomfort so significantly that the mind chatter was reduced as well. I was left with silence. Silence and my surroundings.

I easily could have filled the silence with alternate distractions: podcasts, music, audiobooks. Instead, I made the tough decision to train without them; my aim was to explore this newfound quiet and alone time fully. I wanted to see if I could pull it off. Could I survive without intentionally filling my head with entertainment and distraction? Could I use this quiet time as an opportunity to think and experience? I was curious to find out if my mind could adapt to slowing down the way my body was.

Slowing down mentally was much more difficult than I had imagined it would be. I still vividly remember many an early morning, exiting my back door at 5:00 a.m. for a three-hour run, those first steps in the dark, my headlamp illuminating a small, uneven space just ahead. I remember the quiet almost as a physical sensation rather than the absence of sounds. The extreme quiet. A quiet that, with three small children, I rarely experienced most days. And I remember the misery, the intense feeling that I would so much rather be back in bed, warm and asleep next to my wife. But then, mere minutes later, the chatter would begin to lose its power, its presence.

As I ran forward, into the quiet dark, a gentle transition to an uncomplicated awareness followed—an awareness first of the silence, then of my surroundings: the temperature, the trees, the road, and the trails. A transition to being there, rather than getting there.

Every day, the world is speeding up. As technology continues to advance, our brains are flooded with constant information, entertainment, and general content. Access to all of these resources has made us much more focused on our goals rather than on the path to achieving them. Often this affects how we approach our exercise and fitness—from HIIT training to CrossFit to power yoga—and the tools we use to maximize our goals: step counting, data gathering, micromanaging. This mindset even bleeds into the terminology we use around fitness: boost your metabolism, burn more fat. The message is always that there is a there, and you can get there fast, whether the claims are for losing twenty pounds in twenty days, gaining six-pack abs, or getting beach-body ready.

Slow down on a trail and the need to get anywhere softens. When you physically slow down on a trail, your mind will slow down with you. On the longer-distance runs, the mind tends to let go, and when it does, it begins to just be. In that state, I found an openness of mind within which ideas would appear. It was as if my mind finally had the room for ideas to enter. Ideas for my podcast and videos, and even song lyrics seemed to charge right on in. In fact, the ideas flowed so freely that I started bringing along a pocket digital recorder to record them along the way; otherwise, I would forget so many by the time I finished.

Rather than react to it, I learned to, in a sense, run alongside the physical "need" to speed up and the mental chatter telling me I should. I found a place of presence and calm. I was active rather than reactive—attentive, not distracted. Soon enough, I noticed that this lesson began to alter and improve my life outside of running. I became better equipped to look for and steal moments of quiet in an otherwise busy, noisy world.

Ultrarunning for Normal People is never about winning a race. It is about the experience of getting there. When Normal People arrive at a race, we are ultra-aware of how much we have already accomplished simply by showing up. I desperately wanted to finish my first ultramarathon, but I was cognizant of the immense amount of personal transformation that had already occurred in me up until the starting gun went off.

Normal People show up knowing full well that, for us, it is actually not a race at all, and it's certainly not about winning anything except perhaps in one sense—winning a Normal Person's life. I arrived on race day having internalized the lesson of slowing down, and I was better for it.

Ultrarunning teaches Normal People to slow down.

To Be Versatile

It is a law of nature we overlook, that intellectual versatility is the compensation for change, danger, and trouble. An animal perfectly in harmony with its environment is a perfect mechanism. Nature never appeals to intelligence until habit and instinct are useless. There is no intelligence where there is no change and no need of change. Only those animals partake of intelligence that have a huge variety of needs and dangers.

— H. G. WELLS

It was a Thursday morning when I was training for my first road marathon, and I arrived to begin that day's run completely unready. It was cold, at least by a Northern California coast's winter standard. And I was tired. That day's workout was an interval run because the training plan in the book said so. Up to this point, my relationship with training plans had been less than stellar. My tendency toward militancy prevented me from ever adapting a training plan to my own needs or circumstances,

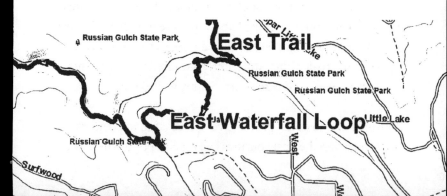

so if a book had "six-mile interval run Thursday" scheduled, I would run the intervals no matter my physical or mental state that day. I often lost myself to the plan. So, that day, off I ran until I ruptured my Achilles tendon.

On the first half mile, I fell and bloodied my knee. I should have turned back right then and there, but instead I pulled myself back up and continued. I managed to get through the interval portion of the run, pushing myself hard because I considered the training plan my coach, the prescribed workout an order. On the last half-mile cooldown, I felt a sudden, painful pop in my left Achilles. Ruptured. I had demanded too much of my body, and it had responded. I hobbled back to my car. I soon found that I could not run for five weeks. So much for militancy.

But not only did the ruptured Achilles prevent me from doing what I wanted to do—run—but it also forced me to contend with my all-or-nothing approach: Was my militancy around training plans serving me? Was I the guy who had to push himself because a book told him to? Or was I the guy who was in charge of his life enough to be versatile and take a day off, especially when his body and mind were screaming at him to? The answer was obvious. The problem was that I had never asked the question until then.

The following year, I dived into the ultramarathon world and read a few ultrarunning books to prepare. I knew that I had much to learn, but one thing I knew for sure was that I did not want to suffer a similar fate as I had during the marathon training. I wanted to do things differently. I wanted to train without injury, train well, and take control of my well-being.

Routines can keep us productive, successful, and on track. However, even the best routines can reach a point where they no longer serve us, and in spite of this, many of us will continue with them because they're what we know. We may think that taking the time to establish a new habit or routine is too daunting and instead stick with what is familiar, comfortable, and known. "Does this routine serve me?" is a surprisingly tough question to ask ourselves, but the answer can be the kick in the ass Normal People need to shake things up and perform better in our lives. If the answer is no, we are faced with two options: one, continue with a routine even though we know it is not good for us; or two, find the strength to replace it by establishing a new one. The second option is ideal, but given how busy and stressed we often are, it is not surprising that most settle by continuing with the same routine. Perhaps the most attractive aspect of our existing routines, regardless of whether they serve us, is that we know them. We're comfortable with them—yes, even the ones that are not making us happy or healthy and perhaps never did. The hard work necessary to improve any aspect of our lives should never be taken lightly, but to evolve we must sometimes change things up, we must learn to become versatile and adaptable. Being versatile, being open to change, has both the power to establish new routines and the power to break them as needed. This is the power of maintaining a higher level of control in our lives—a control I had not had when I ruptured my Achilles. I considered the training routine as the final word, and I felt I had no say in the matter.

One of the things I love about trails is that they embody versatility. You cannot run like a robot on trails. They are naturally uneven, rough, rocky, root-y, hilly, wet, and holey. Trails are perfect in their imperfection, but to run effectively on them, a Normal Person must match the imperfection with the ability to adjust, adapt, change tactics, and improvise at any given moment. The nature of trails can cause even the most well-planned race to go off the rails, and this is something for which a Normal Person must face in virtually any ultramarathon.

Despite plenty of evidence to the contrary these days, I believe human beings are versatile by nature. But in this world, most of us settle into a level of routine and regularity that quite often remains relatively unchanged for most of our lives. We get very used to our regular manner of doing things, thus becoming addicted to the comfort that this regularity affords us. Because most of us know exactly where our next meal is coming from, where we are going to sleep tonight, and how to negotiate the constraints and demands of our jobs and of modern society—how to get places, how to access information—we do not have a real need for significant versatility. We can rely on what we know, and rarely do we have much need to change things up.

However, versatility is in us.

We have the capacity to be surprisingly comfortable with discomfort and change. Our bodies and minds are wired to adapt and adjust, to deal with and survive all that nature presents us with: weather, predators, terrain, caloric scarcity.

Yet our powerful brains continue to put forth systems and technologies that promote and allow comfort, militancy, rigidity, and such strict routines that it is as if we are trying to force the versatility right out of us. But the versatility is there. It may be deep down in the minds of many, but the fact that it is there creates a conflict between our true nature and how we are living our lives.

We must bring out and embrace versatility—both mentally and physically—if we are to effectively train for and finish an ultramarathon. Training solely on a treadmill, a Normal Person will have to endure the inevitable struggle that awaits us when we take our first step onto the perfectly imperfect trails. Treadmills are essentially electric roads, and roads are unnaturally flat, manicured, smooth, and so artificially perfect that our natural, wild human design wants nothing to do with them. For years, we've lived in and around roads, but we still have not adapted to them. Their regularity may render any real need to be versatile useless, but versatility is the very trait that yields success on trails.

I discovered how valuable it is to be versatile while training for two different ultramarathons: my *first* ultramarathon and my *best* ultramarathon.

In preparing for my first ultramarathon, I began working with Flaherty for just the first few months with the intention of getting pointed in the right direction. Together we established a training strategy and basic tenets: to work toward slowing down, to incorporate strength training, and to get in some long hikes. Off I went.

One of the core tenets of training for a trail race is to mix things up, which entails running on trails whenever possible, incorporating some strength training to develop muscles not significantly engaged on roads (like the inside and outside muscles of our legs), and including interval-type runs, in which the trainee alternates fast and slow pacing or hills and downhills. In other words, it's important to make the training irregular and versatile. This is what Flaherty taught me right out of the chute (and what I learned yet again during my training to become a running coach), and I followed the week's plan as he had laid it out for me. However, there was a meta level of versatility on the horizon, a versatility hovering above the variety of the runs, that became one of the biggest lessons I would soon learn.

Some weeks in on the training, Jeff Stanford (co-owner of the resort whose wellness center I help direct) and I were asked to give a series of talks at Beloit College in Wisconsin. The hitch was that Flaherty had set that week's training plan well in advance of the trip, and I was worried about how I would get it done in an unfamiliar location and with a busy travel schedule. I was still hanging on to the idea that the plan was in charge of me and not the other way around. I had to contend with the flights, staying in a hotel, navigating an unfamiliar city, sharing a car, and the possibility that there were no trails close by. All these factors seemed to point to the fact that executing the miles in my training plan was going to be a logistical challenge. Fairly stressed out by the whole prospect, I reached out to Flaherty, assuming I was in for a world of maps, planning, and scheduling. To my surprise, his response was "Fine, just do what you can." In other words, he instructed me not to sweat the existing week's plan and to instead play it by ear. He made quick edits on the week's runs, added an additional day off, and that was that. A simple solution but one that was extremely difficult for me to process.

How foreign a concept, to be able to effortlessly change the plan, to be told so nonchalantly to just do what I could in the middle of training for a fifty-mile trail ultramarathon, while suggesting that doing so would have no negative impact on the outcome. This was a level of embracing versatility that was way bigger than training for an ultramarathon. Though I now believe humans are wired for versatility, I was one human who was living a life far offtrack from accepting my own, and I was a little shocked by such an abrupt and effortless shift on Flaherty's part.

Nevertheless, he was the expert, and I the novice, so I chose to trust him and the process. I proceeded with his revised and less substantial weekly plan. I played it by ear and even made some adjustments of my own. Rather than expending the additional mental energy the original plan would have required—determining the routes in an unfamiliar location and planning the logistics of food and water bottles—I leisurely ran around the college campus and town. Instead of focusing so much on training, I ran with an exploratory mindset of embracing adventure. I ran for fun, *during* my training for a fear-inducing ultramarathon. The versatility that Flaherty had infused in the process granted me a respite, and I enjoyed the Wisconsin runs far more than I would have had I forced myself to push through the original week's plan. In effect, Flaherty's adjustment relegated the training to more of a bonus in the week, instead of what would have been an all-consuming priority. Pushing through with the original plan would have been stress-inducing enough to negatively impact the talks I was giving and my enjoyment of the trip. A Normal Person considers all of this. It is not and can never be 100 percent about the training. We have other fish to fry.

Looking back, I acknowledge that adjusting the plan did not seem to adversely affect my performance on race day. If somehow it did, it made no difference to me because I achieved what I had set out to do: finish and finish well. I have witnessed again and again since then that a few days off here or there during training never makes much difference. This experience was a glimpse into a freedom of mind within which I could see great possibility for my life in general. It was a glimpse into an ability to be versatile enough to accept change, to be able adjust on the fly, and to be in charge of managing my stress better, living my life more fully, and broadening my focus into multiple areas of my life.

Clearly, the versatility of training did not *hurt* me. Rather, I wondered, "Could it have actually helped?"

A year later, I decided to put this question to the test. In 2016, I signed up for the North Face Endurance Challenge 50K and decided to conduct an experiment. I wanted to see how successful (Normal Person success—finishing strong, recovering well, and having fun) I would be with these self-imposed rules and guidelines in place:

I would neither create nor follow any set training plan.

I would neither create nor follow any set nutrition plan on training runs (i.e., no set plan on what or when I ate).

I would show up to the starting line with zero knowledge of the racecourse and no sense for what I would be facing regarding elevation, terrain, or the aid station locations and offerings.

I would show up to the starting line equipped with merely one handheld bottle of water and nothing else—no backpack, gels, sports drink powder, bandages, or extra socks.

In other words, I would fly blind, but I would fly blind on—and with—purpose.

Contrary to how I might have felt at earlier moments in my running career, taking this approach didn't feel like asking for punishment. I'd already experienced running and training for ultra-distances, and I'd already run two trail ultramarathons. I no longer felt the pressure to finish or the fear of not finishing that I'd felt before my first race. Now, when I coach runners, I teach versatility and that mid-training breaks can be beneficial.

However, I do not recommend my particular experiment's level of free-for-all to any novice ultrarunner. Having some planning and structure in place for a first race can build confidence and alleviate some of the fear. For me, however, if this experiment failed, it would just be a lesson learned, incurred with very little cost. I was also traveling to the race with my two training partners, both Normal People themselves: Brie, who was running the race, and Cyd, who was there to cheer us on. If all went to hell, I would drop out mid-race and still have a fun trip with two good friends.

My goal with this new approach was to find out if removing all structure, militancy, and rigidity could deliver me a good race day. In other words, if I approached this race first and foremost from a place of versatility—training more by feel and attempting to integrate it within the context of my family, work, and general schedule—could I achieve a similar outcome as I had for previous races when I militantly followed a plan on the page and significantly moved parts of my life aside to train? And, furthermore, if this versatility actually meant I ran less mileage overall, what would be the outcome? Would I toe the line completely ill prepared? Would this experiment be a recipe for disaster?

We often forget that training—and exercise in general, for that matter—is added stress on our bodies and minds. However, when this stress is constrained to manageable levels, it can actually strengthen us. But it *is* crucial for Normal People to always remember that training is a stressor so that we—as individuals with multiple areas of focus, responsibilities, and obligations—can prevent the quantity and quality of our training from becoming *too* stressful. When we pull this off, most of the time we will escape potential damage to our physical and mental well-being.

Often during ultramarathon training, people incorrectly assume that because they are exercising so much more, they can be more relaxed about what they eat. In fact, the opposite is true.

An apt analogy is to think of our bodies as cars and then to imagine that we decide to run our engines extra hard for the next six months—pedal to the metal. Furthermore, we've decided that *because* we are pushing our vehicles this hard, we do not need to be as concerned about how much oil or how clean the oil is in our engines. While our cars need only gas to run, they need motor oil to run well. Having sufficient and high-quality oil is absolutely essential to the health and function of the cars. Oil is what minimizes the wear and tear and enables our engines to continue burning gas without burning out.

Likewise, our bodies have a greater chance of surviving and even performing well under significant stress when we provide them with the proper nutrients found in healthy food: vitamins, minerals, phytochemicals, antioxidants, and fiber—our bodies' motor oil. The elements of proper nutrition are either absent or nearly absent in unhealthy food. The body, amid the stress of training, which includes the inevitable anxiety and worry about the race (especially for a first ultramarathon), begs us for more and better nourishment. If we ignore our bodies and consume unhealthy food during training, we pile stress on top of stress. This decision can be a recipe for disaster for Normal People—a decision that will affect not only the training itself but also the non-training-related parts of our lives. We could find ourselves less productive at work, more irritable with our families, more fatigued, and more anxious.

The big question is "What constitutes a healthy amount of training stress?" And this is where versatility is essential. A healthy amount is what I refer to in my book *Six Truths* as "the

Goldilocks of stress"—not too much, not too little. While this may sound simple enough, it can be quite complicated when we understand a very important truth:

Normal People do not exercise or train in a vacuum. Normal People train while we live our normal lives. We do not quit our jobs or leave our families to train. We train and we work and we spend time with our families and friends and we continue with our hobbies and interests.

We don't return from a training run and take off the rest of the day, absconding our other responsibilities. We return, take the kids to school, then head off to work. With all of life's other duties, achieving sufficient recovery time can be a tall order. Additionally, we don't have a nutritionist or chef preparing healthy meals for us, and we don't have a coach getting us out the door in the morning or reminding us to take it easy. My own coach, Matt Flaherty, coached me from afar via Google Sheets and some phone calls—ne'er a wake-up call.

Versatility plays a crucial role in our ability to maintain a healthy level of stress. Allowing ourselves to be versatile means we learn to adjust our training based on the entirety of our lives and continue to make large and small adjustments throughout. When something occurs in our normal lives that is a significant enough disruption to our normal routines, we adapt, just as I adapted when Flaherty adjusted my training week due to a temporary disruption with my trip to Wisconsin. The ability to be versatile means not being lured into a book's training regimen that may or may not be appropriate for a given Normal Person's lifestyle. There are not usually wide variations from training plan to training plan, but there is one thing they all have in common: they do not know you personally. Training plans are generalized; they are not customized to your schedule, your responsibilities, or your obligations. In just the few months I worked with Flaherty, I learned to customize my training as needed. While very difficult at first, it has steadily become much easier, and I've found it to be beneficial on every level. Being versatile improved my training, my level of stress, and my life in general.

In the months leading up to the North Face Endurance Challenge 50K, I ran when I could, and I did not when I could not. I ran shorter distances on busier days, longer distances on lighter days, and varied distances based on how I felt. I ate peanut butter and jelly sandwiches on some runs, dried dates on others, gels on still others, and absolutely nothing on quite a few. I drank plain water on some runs, coconut water with goji berries on others, and nothing on quite a few. I intentionally mixed things up and operated by feel. Surprisingly, I had fun with it. There is a lightness and an energy that come with calling our own shots.

Most plans and coaches will tell you to put in around thirty to sixty miles per week while training for a 50K. Some approaches argue for significantly more, others a bit less. However, most hover around that mark, and the weekly mileage typically increases throughout the training period and is broken up by a couple taper weeks. These are weeks during which training requires significantly less mileage, offering a brief physical and mental break, often with the first smack-dab in the middle of training and the second in the week leading up to the race. However, during my experiment, I never surpassed thirty miles per week, and I managed only one long run during the entire training period—a single seventeen-miler that I ran by mistake.

That day, my plan was to run about eleven miles with Cyd and Brie on one of our favorite trails—a trail that is part of the course of the race I direct. About seven miles in, Brie's hip started to give her some hassle, and since she lived nearby, she peeled off. At about ten miles in, Cyd left to get ready for work. Now running solo, I decided to put in another mile or two before calling it a day. That was until I proceeded to get lost. After finishing the water and food I had brought with me—that day's non-preplanned food was a single peanut butter and jelly sandwich—and with no familiar terrain in sight, I finally gave up and texted Brie and Cyd in hopes that they might guide me home. I finally managed to find a signal, a tall order on Mendocino coast trails, and asked for help. Within about a minute, I received the following text messages, in this order:

Brie: Let me know if you can get to anything at all familiar and I'll come back in and get you.

And then, a few seconds later . . .

Cyd: You do realize you got lost on your own racecourse. Fail. Hahahahahahaha.

Thankfully, I made it out and back home without too much trouble, but such is the world of trail running. In training for that race, I ran significantly fewer miles, and, ultimately, it did not seem to have much of a bearing on the outcome. But there was another significant piece of this experiment that made the training atypical for me: I did not *only* run. I was shown the profound value of versatility yet again.

Six months prior to toeing the line at the North Face Endurance Challenge 50K, I had completed a ten-week course taught by Wim Hof, a multiple world-record-holder and practitioner of extreme physical feats. The Wim Hof Method®, which he argues keeps the body and mind operating optimally in its natural state, is essentially a combination of a breathing technique, meditation, and cold therapy, plus a yoga practice integrated with breath. No longer militantly following a formal 50K training plan, I had more time and energy to explore another training modality, and I entered an entirely different and unfamiliar world. Suddenly, I found myself in daily cold showers and rounds of Wim's breathwork technique. Admittedly, I did not begin the course with the intention of enhancing my training or with any idea that the breathwork and cold therapy would have any effect on my experiment, much less a profound effect. I began it simply because I had the time and the interest, so I forged ahead.

As with ultrarunning, I entered into cold therapy and this particular breathwork method with some trepidation. Yet again I was embarking into uncharted territory but with less fear—though the cold therapy is no walk in the park—and my efforts certainly yielded unforeseen benefits. Each day, I completed at least four rounds of Wim Hof breathing.

A single round goes as follows:

Take thirty to forty deep, fairly rapid breaths
(breathing fully in and then releasing the exhale
fully out but not pushing it out). This acts as an intentional
and focused hyperventilation that triggers stress and
hormonal responses in the body but without any perceived
danger or threat typically present when hyperventilating.

Release the breath in a final exhalation until it stops
by itself (i.e. again, refraining from pushing out).

Hold there (on the exhale) until you
feel the need to breathe.

Inhale fully and holding this inhale for
about ten to fifteen seconds.

Release the breath.

Once a round is completed, you launch into the next and repeat until you have completed four or more rounds. Senses become increasingly heightened during the rounds, and one often feels tingling sensations and sees various lights or flashes with closed eyes. The quickened breathing and subsequent hold on the exhale exercise the cardiovascular system by bringing in slightly more oxygen and expelling a ton of carbon dioxide, which allows a slow build of carbon dioxide during the held exhale that first constricts then dilates the blood vessels. In addition, the heart rate fluctuates during the hyperventilation period and the subsequent rest while holding the breath.

The most rewarding feeling during the rounds is the sense of total relaxation while holding the exhale. During this hold, which can last up to three minutes by the fourth round, there is virtually no muscular contraction (unlike the effort it takes to hold an inhale). You have just relaxingly released the exhale until it stops by itself—what I call hitting the "natural bottom." This relaxation is full and unparalleled; at no other time is the body at that level of stillness. This breathing technique is fairly well studied, with more research ongoing.

The accompanying cold therapy, while part of the Wim Hof Method®, is a very different experience than the breathwork. Cold therapy is definitely my "do one thing that scares you every day" activity. It is a daily dose of fear, dread, discomfort, and challenge. It is an exercise of mind over matter and requires a focused effort to calm and relax. The breath is the portal to that calm. Controlling my breath means controlling my stress. When getting into the cold—an ice bath, a cold shower, or the ocean—I do some breathwork and enter the water relaxed, with none of the quick, panicked inhales one usually experiences when getting in extremely cold water. I stay in for two to five minutes, and after the first thirty seconds or so, I feel surprisingly fine, cold on the outside but warm internally. A side effect of both breathwork and cold therapy is an increased awareness of the body, a phenomenon referred to as "interoception." Put simply, in moments of presence and awareness, we notice more. Make no mistake, however—the first thirty seconds has never been pleasurable or comfortable. It has, 100 percent of the time, been dreadful. But that is the point: to move through the fear and coexist with the discomfort.

The breathing, cold therapy, mindset, yoga, and running improved my endurance, fitness, race-day performance, and postrace recovery. A versatile and varied approach to self-care, stress, and training is vital to a Normal Person's success. Following previous ultras, I would be sore and limping for several days, but this time was different. This time, though I certainly refrained from doing so, I could have run the very next day. My wife remarked, "You don't seem that sore." And I wasn't.

What was it that yielded a positive race-day outcome? Was it the yoga, the breathing, the cold, the less overall mileage, purposefully mixing up the training food? In hindsight, I believe it was a combination of everything. But perhaps an even more accurate assessment was the general mindset that empowered me to embrace those individual factors. Perhaps the day was successful because I'd had to adopt a versatile mindset, a mindset that freed me to adjust my training and enabled me to diversify it. With this freedom, I became more effective at maintaining my overall stress as it related to both my body and mind. I improved and strengthened by making sure to push myself *just enough*, and not just in one area. This time around, the amount of stress seemed to have been just right, not because I finished under a certain time or set a personal record but because I had a great experience and learned a ton and because I did not have to make major life adjustments to have the experience I had.

The science of stress and its effects on the body, both positive and negative, is well researched, and this time I had used stress to my advantage. Looking back, I realized not only that I had been overtraining for my previous races but that I had also made the training almost entirely running focused. Finally, I had learned not to make that mistake. This time, with this experiment, I showed up to the starting line as a stronger runner and a stronger human being.

In this, as with the other lessons I've learned from ultrarunning, I made the connection to the rest of my Normal Person's life. My newfound versatility and adaptability in the training arena spilled over into all areas of my life, and, to this day, it serves me as a person, not just a runner.

Ultrarunning teaches Normal People to be versatile.

To Pay Attention in Everything

Pay attention. It's all about paying attention.
Attention is vitality. It connects you with others.
It makes you eager. Stay eager.

— SUSAN SONTAG

Many trails are narrow, and some are a single track, with no room for anyone to run next to you. This terrain sets trail running apart from road races in a profound way. Showing up to any race is often, at least in part, a social decision. Humans crave social interaction and thrive with it. We value shared experiences, and running races of all distances delivers this. From a social standpoint, road races are superior to races on single-track trails. On roads, participants can run next to friends, family, and groups of strangers. We will value anyone we can hang out with and with whom we can pass the time during a race. We welcome distraction from struggle and discomfort, and in a race where physical limits are tested, there is nothing better than running alongside people who can take our minds off the pain.

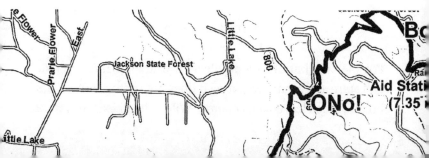

I experienced this firsthand during my two road marathons. Surrounded by groups of runners for the entire race, I chatted, joked, struggled, complained, listened to others complain, supported, received support, and felt a palpable comradery with the other runners. Every single one of these interactions was a boon to the overall experience. They made the time and the miles go by faster, all while mitigating the discomfort. The comradery alone explains the draw for road races.

Though there is a social aspect and benefit of trail ultramarathons, they are quite different than road races. Ultramarathoners are a tight-knit community, partly due to the fact that it is still a comparatively small sport. But races are social by nature, whether they're run on road or trail. There is always the possibility of training with friends, the fun time spent together pre- and postrace, and all the talk between runners leading up to the race. Though trail ultras diverge from road races at the exact point in a trail ultramarathon at which the course narrows to a single-track trail. At this point, the group experience largely disappears, and we are suddenly and rather abruptly left alone. We are left with only ourselves to feel and hear—the voice in our heads—and with hopefully a grounded faith and hope that our training will get us through all the unknowns that are sure to come.

But at that point, on a narrow trail of dirt and rocks, we are faced with yet another reality. A reality that is foreign to most Normal People but very familiar to those who become trail ultrarunners.

Forced attention.

For me, meditation is a privilege. A wild animal doesn't sit and stare at a candle or statue; it does not try to "witness" its breath, much less chant a mantra. Wild animals exist in a state of attention because their survival depends on it. They constantly watch, look, and listen. They are always paying attention, and this state is integrated into their lives. Humans, on the other hand, can sit. At least those of us who can afford to, and by that, I mean those of us whose circumstances, financial and otherwise, afford us an ability to periodically check out from the world. Even Tibetan monks who meditate all day do so in or around the safety of a building, with a kitchen (and someone else to prepare their food), a restroom, and a roof. Most meditators do their business in a relatively quiet, temperature-controlled, comfortable, and safe place.

In this way, meditation is much like exercise. Wild animals do not exercise. They do not get on a treadmill and go nowhere for forty-five minutes, much less for the purpose of increasing cardiovascular health, lowering their resting heart rate, burning more calories, avoiding diabetes, or increasing their maximal oxygen consumption (VO_2 max). Instead, wild animals just *move*, and their movement is integrated into their lives. They move to find food, to escape danger, and to find shelter. Just as with being in a state of attention, their survival depends on movement. Humans, on the other hand, do exercise. We are the only species that moves for no immediate survival-based reason, sometimes for a relatively short period of time. Then, for the rest of our day, we are often shockingly sedentary. In fact, basic survival in the modern world requires very little movement at all—food delivery services, cars, planes, and even electric walkways in our airports have all but erased any real need to move our bodies to ensure our survival.

Trail running forces attention, a type I refer to as "wild attention." Wild attention combines movement and meditation in a way that most other sports do not. Some refer to this as "active meditation." And while our survival does not depend on running trails, the experience of being alone on a trail is a pretty accurate simulation of our wilder days—days when humans were forced by survival to be in a state of attention and to move.

Training for my first ultramarathon and having had discovered trail running only a short time prior, I was struck by a more effortless awareness and attention than I had ever known. Of course, as with any form of meditation, my mind would wander, but only for a few moments before effortlessly returning to the task at hand: negotiating the trails, staying upright, and scanning the feet ahead for obstacles. The trail brought me back to the present. Usually. Longer bouts of daydreaming (more frequent in the early days on trails) would inevitably result in a good, hard fall or, at minimum, a toe-bruising stumble—the physical cost of losing focus for just one moment too long. A trail's demand of wild attention manifests in the form of rocks, roots, ups, downs, turns, poison oak, stinging nettles, wild animals, and more. Lose focus and one or more of these will take you down. In fact, one of my knees has permanent scar tissue from repeated tumbles on the exact same place on my body. Apparently, I have a distinct and specific way of falling—a pair of sweatpants with a hole in that exact spot is further proof.

Having experienced wild attention for the first time on the trails while training for the fifty-miler, I now know that I wasn't just training physically; I was training mentally. The uneven and unpredictable terrain, increased distances, and lengthier durations converged to increase and improve my mental focus and toughness, even though I never set out with the intention to improve either. As the quantity of my runs progressed—and with them, my physical fitness—I noticed not only an increased calming of my mind but also a greater awareness of my surroundings.

Ultrarunning was training me to open my awareness window. No longer fixated on a singular focus—a statue, a candle, the sound of my breath—I was learning to broaden the scope of my awareness, to listen, look, and feel everything, all at once.

Many artists describe receiving inspiration as if it originated from somewhere outside of them. I have experienced this phenomenon many times on trails, when in a state of wild attention, one of the many positive side effects of this mindset. Ideas for books, podcasts, videos, and even song lyrics would come, and they still do. In effect, the combination of solitude and quiet creates a space for ideas to appear. Where they come from is inconsequential. Perhaps they are already there but the noise that fills our heads most of the time acts as a wall that keeps ideas, inspiration, and passion from reaching us. In wild attention, they all get through, they show up. That they show up in this context is what makes trail running so valuable for Normal People.

So plentiful were the ideas that came to me on the trails that very soon I began carrying a small pocket-size digital recorder to document the ideas as they arrived. Prior to documenting them, I would forget most by the time I returned, especially on the three- or four-hour training runs. I'd often return home with multiple ideas on the recorder; some I'd keep, some I'd delete, but the influx occurred either way.

Clients often tell me that they are searching for inspiration, for something about which they can feel passionate. My advice is that they should actively pursue neither. Instead, I steer them to actions that lead to moments of solitude and personal quiet devoid of any intentional noise they might be shoving into their own heads. I refer to this process as "stealing moments" because the pull of distraction, and even our obligations and responsibilities, is so intense that it takes a focused, intentional effort to grab even a semblance of quiet. The demands of the modern world make it such that we are forced to steal the time we need to think and process. Making the conscious move to hit a trail checks all the boxes: solitude, quiet, attention. In other words, I advise Normal People to focus their efforts not on finding passion but rather on creating an environment that will facilitate the arrival of inspiration. Trails are the perfect environment for this.

For years now, I have been creating content: almost four hundred podcast episodes, nearly three hundred YouTube videos, hundreds of songs, and four books. Trail running became an unexpected work tool for me. It has substantially decreased the amount of time and effort I need to come up with ideas for content. I have always tried to avoid forcing this process or creating content for content's sake, choosing instead to put something in the world only when it is important enough for me to do so. At the time of this writing, I have finished recording my first new album in over fifteen years, and some of the lyrics for the songs even came to me on the trails. Our individual inspirations are only the tip of the iceberg of what we can "hear" when in an environment that quiets the chatter in our heads enough for us to listen.

Ultrarunning does a bang-up job of getting us to a place of quiet. For me, a long trail run is a series of stolen moments chained together in a lengthy string of time. A little distraction, back to the present, a little distraction, back to the present, and so forth. But by their nature, the trails aid each return to the present. To the outside world, it may look like exercise, but to the Normal Person, running on a single-track trail is a quiet, a silence, and a nod to what it takes to keep ourselves grounded in an otherwise floaty world. On a trail, we are in our time, our space, and we are able to silence a chattering mind.

Glimpses of wild attention come immediately, but our ability to channel improves over time. Most Normal People are quite used to being inundated with all the noise. So much so that when we find ourselves in relative quiet, it can be very unsettling. There is a detox of sorts that occurs on the trails, which means that Normal People can reasonably expect some restlessness in the beginning. This often results in loud mind chatter and an intense craving for distraction. That's the bad news. The good news is that it gets better because we adapt. And when we adapt, we get better. Our minds settle over time, and eventually we crave the calm. We crave it because within this calm we take notice of what we have in our lives, and we are thankful for it. Creating this environment of calm is easier said than done—it is all too easy to say the words "live in gratitude," but to truly reach this place is worth it.

> *In wild attention, time changes—or, more specifically, our perception of time alters.*

In our distraction-based world, time seems to move very quickly, but out on trails, especially as we inch toward the longer distances, it feels slower. Add in the inevitable discomfort that increases along with the distance, and we are nudged into even greater presence and awareness, an even slower perception of time. On a trail, it is nearly impossible to be distracted for any significant amount of time. We are forced to pay attention in the truest sense of the phrase. This attention is a currency we trade for a more fulfilling life, a life lived on our terms, a life that allows for and even embraces discomfort and pain so that we may acquire a fuller experience of joy.

If there is a downside to paying more attention, it is that in doing so, we are increasingly confronted with the parts of us and our lives from which we have been distracting ourselves. So, in moments of awareness, of wild attention, we are confronted and wrestle with our so-called flaws and mistakes. In these moments, we do not practice shutting off. We do not hide. We see.

In my coaching work, I ask my clients to clearly define and describe their most ideal lives as if they were already living them: what kind of relationship they are in, what job they have, where they live, what kind of house they live in, what their relationship to food is like, how well they treat themselves and others, what they do creatively. In doing this exercise, they see a picture of their own ideals—and perhaps on some level how they already see themselves. I believe the struggles with health and happiness that exist for many are about not becoming someone new but rather working to bring our already-existing ideals into the world. The first step is to identify where conflicts exist—incongruities between how we have been acting in our lives and our ideals. For example, some overweight clients write that in their ideal life they are at a healthy weight. Some self-described bingers write that in their ideal life they have a healthy relationship with food and do not overeat. These ideals define them. In fact, in my second book, about healthy and happy families, I wrote about how I resolved my own conflict between my reality of coming in the house at the end of the day, glued to my phone, and my ideal of coming in, setting my phone on the counter, and being present with my family.

This process is about acknowledging that how we have been behaving may not be who we really are. By discovering what we really stand for and value, we are liberated from defining ourselves by how we might have been living, which in turn allows us to begin the hard work of living more fully as our true selves. Instead of the damaging, harsh narrative of "I'm just a binger. I have no self-control, it's just who I am," through this exercise, that same individual can frame it this way: "Yes, I have been binging for years, but it is not who I am. Now that I know who I am, I can begin the process of bringing the real me into the world." Defining our ideals gives us a direction in which to move our lives. It grounds us and frees us.

Becoming aware of these conflicts is never pleasant, which is why we take advantage of every opportunity to distract ourselves. But by identifying which of our actions do not serve us and, more importantly, how the ideal version of ourselves would act, we empower ourselves to immediately begin moving in the direction of a happier, healthier life. We have to first know where we are going in order to get there. In my work, I refer to this approach as "mind first, body second." Do the thinking, earn the mindset, and then begin to move. A Normal Person on a trail can achieve this; we can access the time and space necessary to think deeply. But make no mistake: this process takes time, awareness, patience, compassion, and attention.

We are imperfect as individuals and as a species. This imperfection is built into our very design. Yet we would rather shut ourselves off to the things in our lives we want to improve than simply set out to improve them. If, however, we desire to live more fully, we must take the good and the bad, the comfortable and the uncomfortable, the beautiful and the ugly. We must accept our imperfections and still work to live closer to our ideals in spite of them. It is not possible to be selectively attentive and turn away only from what we do not want to see. Happiness and fulfillment do not work that way, and any attempt to filter out the bad will require more and more distraction. Enter drugs, alcohol, junk food, and social media.

Opening our lives to wild attention, as incredible and powerful as it is, can take it out of us. We need recovery time from this mindset just as we do from the trails. Normal People deserve breaks. Sometimes we need to check out. We need distractions from time to time. But in a state of paying attention in our lives, the purpose of these breaks is not to hide, not to escape what we long to improve, but rather to make the choice to blow off some steam now and then—to have fun, hang out with friends, travel, eat some junk food. The difference is action rather than reaction. Being truly attentive simply means controlling the quantity and frequency of our distractions instead of being controlled by them. We are in charge of when, how, and where we engage in distraction. We learn to seek distraction as a choice, and we come to know when it is necessary. Nevertheless, the background of a successful life is attention. Authentic attention is attention to everything. It does not discriminate. True attention is capital A Attention. It requires constant, challenging work and is not some self-help mindfulness fluff. Attention must never be partitioned. We are either paying attention (to everything), or we are not.

In wild attention, we allow ourselves to feel. We cease to overthink, overanalyze, overprocess.

And then we feel, and exist in feeling, much more than we do while living our regular, normal lives. With practice and continued, intentional forays onto the trails, Normal People find it increasingly easier to notice and accept all the truths of our lives—even the hard ones.

Trail ultrarunning trains Normal People for this level of attention. While it is our choice to run on trails, we do not decide when the trails put us in a state of presence and awareness. Very quickly, the trails teach us the ability to act *and* react at the same time. We learn to notice. While in wild attention, we learn that pain and beauty can exist simultaneously. The trail coaxes us into an attentive state. The trail, with its uneven terrain, bumps, roots, grooves, and rocks, takes us there. The surroundings—the trees, sky, weather, animals, plants, and air—keep us there. When we are running on trails, we—in a profoundly incredible way—have no choice in the matter. And then, something great happens: the attention we pay on the trails effortlessly transitions to our non-trail-running lives. We find ourselves paying greater attention in all that we do, on and off the trail.

*Ultrarunning teaches Normal People
to pay attention in everything.*

To Breathe

We live most life, whoever breathes most air.

— ELIZABETH BARRETT BROWNING

I took all of one history class in college. History was not my bag, but I needed to take the class to satisfy my general education requirements. I have since come to appreciate the subject, but back then, it seemed a rather senseless act of memorizing dates and events, then regurgitating them. I was a philosophy major and preferred laboring over a single paragraph in a Kant manifesto to documenting some battle's timeline. Fearing a bad grade in the class, I opted to switch the class to a "Pass/Fail," which shows up on your transcript as a "Pass," if you get at least a D, and therefore does not affect your GPA. However, I did better than I expected, earning a B+, but in doing so, I wasted one of my Pass/Fail opportunities. I worked hard in the class and learned something, but if not for one standout moment, the experience would most likely have passed me by. The moment—something very unique and unrelated

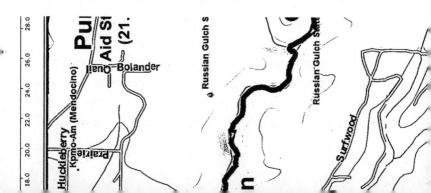

to history—occurred the day of finals. Mere seconds before the class began writing the final exam essays, I encountered a moment I have never forgotten and that has taken me years to fully appreciate.

I vividly remember heading into class that day, finding a seat toward the back of the large auditorium, and opening my floppy blue notebook. Someone handed me the essay questions, then the professor uttered a simple, terse statement.

"Remember to breathe."

At the time, I thought that statement was about as ridiculous as the course itself, and rather pointless. Remember to breathe? As if breathing wasn't biologically obligatory. We do it automatically. Yet years later I came to profoundly appreciate the professor's simple directive, just as I did the subject of history. I now believe it was a piece of crucial wisdom—wisdom most likely overlooked and underappreciated by all the undergrads sitting there in that lecture hall.

In the summer of 2017, I began the Wim Hof ten-week course and launched into a daily practice of the breathing exercise we touched on in the previous chapter, plus cold therapy and a light yoga practice. What I appreciated about Wim Hof, and what convinced me to tackle his course in the first place, was his claim that he could teach anyone his approach. In other words, he was not claiming to be some keeper of magic superpowers that only he was blessed with (what I call in *Six Truths* the "subtle cult"). He has repeatedly offered himself up to science, and he has been studied by major universities. While research is still somewhat in its infancy, the results thus far are exciting: breakthroughs on stress (especially hormetic stress), depression, control over the autonomic nervous system, inflammation, the body's adaptive ability, and more.

Since completing the course over five years ago, I've practiced the breathing technique and cold therapy nearly every single day. I've explored numerous ways to access cold therapy, from cold showers and soaks in my local river and the Pacific Ocean to ice baths. I've embraced it so much (and in order to save some water) I purchased a cold tub that circulates the water and maintains it at a steady thirty-nine degrees Fahrenheit—picture a jacuzzi but super cold and for crazy-but-still-mostly-Normal People.

Over the years, I have dabbled in various breathing techniques both as part of and independent of meditation. As with most healthy acts—engaging in exercise, cold therapy, sauna, meditation, journaling, and proper nutrition—the various breathing approaches are meaningless unless one makes the time and effort to develop them into an actual practice. At least in part as a result of adopting a versatile approach to my training, I developed the Wim Hof Method into a consistent, daily habit rather effortlessly. Fairly quickly, I noticed mental and physical improvements, both of which helped to further cement the practice into my life.

Not long after completing the Wim Hof course, I toed the line at the North Face Endurance Challenge 50K with the self-imposed experiment described in lesson three. Along with the intentional unknown of it all, I decided to use the breathing technique during the race (albeit devoid of Hof's signature breath holds on the exhales, so just the fully-in, let-go approach to breathing). I practiced the breath during most of the race, and when I felt especially fatigued, I would pause, stand still, and continue the breathing until I regained strength, at which point

I would proceed. On a few of those breaks, runners came up to me and said something along the lines of "You can do it!" or "Are you okay?" Both sentiments were at once appreciated and mildly annoying. "I'm fine," I replied. "Just catching my breath." Off they went, then off I went.

While I believe my success on that race day and my speedy recovery after were a result of multiple factors, the breathwork was definitely one of them. I used that experience as an impetus and inspiration to turn the Wim Hof Method into a daily practice. It was my first real experience with incorporating breathwork as a way to regulate stress, especially when faced with the inordinate amount of stress that an ultramarathon necessitates. There is the stress we choose to take on (the ultramarathon) and the stress that we accept as part of our lives (our work, finances, family obligations), and there is the unexpected (a car accident, sickness). Breathwork does an amazing job of helping us get through all of these.

I now practice two types of breathwork: the Wim Hof Method and Oxygen Advantage®. Both have their benefits and specific applications, and while there is some crossover, the two are quite distinct in their methods and goals.

I see and use the Wim Hof Method as a workout session, complete with a start time and an end time. Altogether, the session usually lasts between twenty and thirty minutes. I perform it once a day, usually in the morning. What is most important to note, however, is that I do not breathe this way—with quick in-and-out breaths through the mouth—at any other time. Wim Hof makes no claim that this technique offers anything remotely related to a functional, regular breathing method—a way for most of us to breathe most of the time. Using his breath technique in our everyday lives would be like going for a run in the morning and then continuing that running pace while working, going to the grocery store, or sleeping. I run for shorter periods of time so that my body and mind are calmer and healthier at all other times. Running is an exercise I do for a certain amount of time during my day until I stop doing it. So, too, are my Wim Hof breathing sessions.

I was fascinated by the world of breathwork and continued researching its effects on the body and mind. It was during this research that I stumbled upon another breathing approach, Oxygen Advantage, and this modality in particular took my training even further. Oxygen Advantage has prescribed exercises, but unlike the Wim Hof Method, its aim is to train the body and mind to functionally breath most times, both while awake and asleep. I was hooked, drawn to an approach that would elicit an improvement in my breathing at all times. While I continued with the Wim Hof Method daily, I began to incorporate the Oxygen Advantage's exercises too. Within weeks, I began to experience a shift in my breathing patterns during exercise, work, free time, and sleep.

Whatever breathing technique one pursues, assuming it is studied and legitimate, its effects should be to achieve all that functional breathing can achieve: decreased inflammation; a more robust immune system; improved sleep, especially deep sleep because quality of sleep is as important, if not more so, as quantity; decreased anxiety; improved endurance; increased fat adaptivity, the body's ability to utilize a greater proportion of fat as energy; and more. Both the Wim Hof Method and Oxygen Advantage have served me well, but I am more focused on improving my (and my clients') most-of-the-time breathing, and I have witnessed the greatest improvements with that focus. For this reason, I became an Oxygen Advantage instructor, and it has taken the pole position in my coaching, even over nutrition and running. I have found that once people are able to breathe functionally, they can manage their stress so effectively that changes in eating and exercise more easily occur. I have seen plenty of clients change their dietary habits—such as improving on stress eating, emotional eating, or overeating—simply by learning to breathe slow and relaxed.

Perhaps surprising to many, ever-increasing daily stress has caused most humans to actually *overbreathe*. We take more breaths per minute (referred to as "per minute ventilation") than is healthy in terms of proper and efficient oxygenation of our tissues. On the surface, it may seem that taking more breaths would be ideal—more oxygen coming in, which in theory should mean more oxygen entering the tissues. But this is actually not the case. In fact, any oxygen deficiencies that may exist in our tissues are most likely not due to insufficient oxygen being inhaled. When measured with a pulse oximeter, most humans have plenty of oxygen in their blood at any given time. The average person's reading will likely fall between 95 to 99 percent blood oxygen saturation. Significantly increasing your per minute ventilation or hyperventilating, as with the Wim Hof Method, will increase this percentage at most by only a few percentage points. So if we are breathing in plenty of oxygen and plenty of it makes it into our blood, then why aren't our tissues sufficiently oxygenated? Surprisingly, the answer isn't about oxygen at all, but rather carbon dioxide—a supposed waste product that we assume is best completely cleared from our bodies. But with a closer eye on carbon dioxide, a very different story about functional breathing and the human body emerges.

Carbon dioxide has multiple functions in the body, but perhaps its most important role has to do with its effect on oxygen in the blood. Carbon dioxide is what triggers the release of oxygen into the tissues. But to trigger this release, carbon dioxide levels must be high enough. So while we must exhale carbon dioxide, breathing functionally means not exhaling too much. Exhaling too much leads to insufficient amounts of carbon dioxide in our blood—not enough to move the oxygen out of the blood and into the tissues. As such, when we overbreathe due to a higher baseline of stress in today's world, taking too many breaths per minute, we are blowing out too much carbon dioxide. The result is that oxygen remains in the blood rather than going where we need it to go. Oddly, most of us need more carbon dioxide in our blood most of the time, not less.

Therefore, to breathe functionally is to decrease the amount of breaths we take per minute so that we decrease the amount of carbon dioxide we are exhaling and allow it to sufficiently build up between breaths. The goal of the approach I teach is to train people to take fewer, slower breaths. Creating a habit of slow breathing—taking fewer breaths per minute—when we are going about the general business of our lives increases the amount of oxygen that gets into our tissues. Creating this habit, like all habits, takes a significant amount of work, practice, and time.

But there is an added challenge beyond merely establishing a practice of breathing lighter and slower, and this has to do with the other significant role carbon dioxide plays in the body: it is not the lack of oxygen that triggers a feeling of needing to breathe, but rather the increase of carbon dioxide. When chemoreceptors in our cardiovascular system sense too much carbon dioxide, a message is sent to the brain that it is time to take a breath. But in slowing our breaths down and thereby allowing more carbon dioxide to build in the bloodstream, we will initially feel a strong "air hunger"—a powerful sense of needing to take a breath. In effect, by our having become chronic overbreathers and blowing out too much carbon dioxide, we are keeping the levels chronically too low, such that we feel the need to breathe long before our carbon dioxide levels are able to rise enough to facilitate greater tissue oxygenation. In other words, we blow out too much carbon dioxide, and it doesn't take much release to cause us to feel the need to breathe. Our higher-than-natural baseline of stress has caused us to adopt a way of breathing that has made us too sensitive to carbon dioxide.

While the solution may sound easy enough—to slow and soften our breathing to allow more carbon dioxide to remain in our bloodstream—the struggle is that even a slight increase in carbon dioxide will initially make us feel as though we are not getting enough oxygen. As a result, the work of any breath approach aimed at training (or retraining) a human being to adopt a functional breathing pattern must utilize tools and exercises that sufficiently desensitize the body to carbon dioxide.

> *To undo the bad breathing habits of the modern world, we must engage in exercises that return us to functional breathing patterns.*

Normal People must understand that there is no hacking this process—it takes time and attention, much like anything we add into our lives with the intention of establishing a true habit around it.

Perhaps what I love most about the Oxygen Advantage breathwork approach, and why I chose to become one of their instructors, is that it is not a new way to breathe but rather a return to a more natural way of breathing. In virtually every area of life, we humans are moving further and further away from what is natural to us: the way we eat, socialize, move, and breathe. Still, moving closer to what is more in line with our physiological and psychological design serves Normal People extremely well—especially Normal People ultrarunners.

So when my history professor said, "Remember to breathe," it was sage advice that has stayed with me. During my experimental 50K, I did just that: I remembered to breathe. I remembered to focus on my breath, albeit through the Wim Hof lens, and to ease up a bit when I felt my breath get away from me. This paid off, so much so that my fitness training since the experiment has shifted to the Oxygen Advantage breathing method. I now use nasal breathing on both inhaling and exhaling with scattered breath holds during workouts, always on the exhale. My attention to and work with my breath has transformed how I live, train, and coach others, much in the same way that nutrition, sleep, fitness, and general stress management has.

For me now, breathing during a history final is as essential as breathing during an ultramarathon. A conscious attention to breath in any context is truly a conscious attention to stress. Keep the stress down, and oxygenation—of all tissues, including the brain—stays up. We are less anxious and stressed, and we think more clearly. By periodically checking in on our breath, we reground and slow down, or at least discover that we need to. It is a habit that pays off in a huge way, and one that affects our behavior in practically every area of our lives. I've worked to slow my breath in my non-training life to about six breaths per minute, with four-second inhales and six-second exhales, very light and soft.

While training, my breathing focus is on maintaining the ability to inhale and exhale solely through my nose. On trails, if I find myself unable to inhale and exhale through my nose, I slow down until I can. The only exceptions are times of acute stress, such as hitting a particularly steep trail or during interval, tempo, or hill training runs, or similar types of workouts on a rower or stationary bike—any times of significant enough increases in intensity and stress. When this intensity increases,

I temporarily transition to mouth breathing and then as soon as possible return to nasal breathing as the stress subsides (e.g., in between the intervals or coming back down from a hill).

Over the last few years, with focused and hard work, I have developed a daily practice and habit of breathwork. While I am driving or working, and even taking meetings, I work to keep my breath relaxed, light, and slow. I feel the benefit of this practice in the quality of my sleep and overall stress. I am less reactive in all areas of my life—during social interactions, at work, and around food. With these noticeable improvements, I am inspired to keep breathwork in my life just as I keep healthy eating and exercise in my life. Each facet is valuable, and each part and parcel of a higher-quality existence for Normal People.

On race day, elite athletes push extremely hard because they are going for the win. So hard, that mouth breathing may be, for them, a physiological necessity. On the other hand, Normal People, whose goals aren't to win the race or even come close, have an opportunity to keep our breathing calm and relaxed and through the nose, not only during training but also throughout much of any ultramarathon we attempt. On trails, how we are breathing can be an effective gauge of how well we are maintaining our stress and, therefore, how effectively we are training. If we are breathing through our noses, we are most likely at a sustainable level of stress—a level that increases our chances of running distances like those in ultramarathons. Yes, Normal People can learn to maintain calm and focus even during the gargantuan feat of a trail ultramarathon and, for that matter, the gargantuan task of living a successful life. In fact, I believe trail ultrarunning, like my history professor, reminds us to breathe.

Ultrarunning teaches Normal People to breathe.

To Always Be in Training

Success usually comes to those who are too busy to be looking for it.

— HENRY DAVID THOREAU

During my fifty-miler, at about mile forty-five, another runner came up alongside me. With only five miles to go, we were both in good moods but fatigued just the same. We got to talking, mostly light conversation and pleasantries. After a few minutes, I bid him farewell, and he continued past me at a pace I could not maintain. As he ran ahead, I noticed something peculiar. This runner was significantly overweight. This was one of the many times I have marveled at the complexity and strength of the human body, while at the same time realizing that health and fitness are not always intertwined. This guy was obviously a better runner than I. His body was more capable than mine, at least on this day, at this race. But his body was sending him a message that all was not well. There was stress on his body that was more than it could handle, an imbalance, and his body was screaming about it.

While it is true that an overweight person can be healthier than a person technically at a "healthy" weight (the BMI chart is not an accurate indicator of health), there is no escaping the fact that carrying extra weight (or being underweight) is a sign that something is amiss—improper nutrition, low quality sleep, inordinate work stress, family stress, economic stress, or a combination of factors. Yet in spite of having a body under stress, this runner was still able to finish a fifty-mile race and finish it well. For me, this was something to behold. There exists a power in the human body so great that an obviously challenging feat of endurance—a fifty-mile trail run with a ton of climb—is achievable even for a body under significant stress.

The question then for me was not "Can it be done?" Clearly, the answer was an undeniable yes, as I watched him saunter on ahead of me. The question now was "Can it be sustained?" With a substandard baseline level of health, can something like an ultramarathon, especially if repeated with some decent measure of frequency, take someone down? I believe the answer is most definitely yes. There is a cost to living with too much stress day-to-day and then, on top of that, adding periodic large spikes of stress, such as ultramarathons. The overall cost is a life negatively affected and unsustainable, including the life we come home to after we cross an ultramarathon finish line.

There is a cost to pushing too hard too often, for elite athletes and Normal People alike.

For me, there is a vast difference between training for a specific race and always being in training. Normal People train for ultramarathons, but because our concerns and interests are so much greater than ultras and certainly not in winning them, we thrive when we bring a training mindset to our non-ultramarathon lives. When we establish a daily habit of training, we build a strong foundation of health, strength, focus, and happiness. A strong aim of managed stress and health applied to our Normal Person lives empowers us to thrive. That foundation is a perfect jumping-off point for us to explore challenges of all kinds—including, of course, ultramarathons. We always train in our lives so that we train better for our ultras.

Most elite athletes have seasons. They have race seasons and game seasons during which they train and train hard. Prior to each season's start, they get in shape and continue the hard work until the season finishes. Then comes the offseason, the season of recovery, and training ceases or, at the very least, decreases. This offseason is crucial to the performance-focused season and provides balance. The training is so intense and focused that an extended downtime is absolutely necessary to facilitate a proper and full recovery. In other words, if the intensity of the on-season training were to continue without a break, these athletes would almost certainly face injury, sickness, or fatigue. Sufficient recovery time is essential, both mentally and physically, which is why elite athletes focus so much effort on building proper recovery into their overall compete-to-win strategy.

Cut to Normal People. We do not have seasons in the same context. We find a race and think, "Yeah, that sounds fun. I'll register for that one." There is no major life shift that follows this decision, nor during the training that ensues. We do not stop taking our kids to school or folding our laundry. We do not quit our jobs, work for hours with a coach every day, or temporarily move to another part of the country to train. We usually do a little research into training plans, then make some relatively minor schedule adjustments over the following weeks to carve out sufficient time in our busy lives to accommodate increases in our exercise regimens. We might even enroll a friend or coworker to train with us to infuse some accountability and fun into the equation. But there is no seismic shift to our day-to-day. Our families are not relegated to the back burner. So, while Normal People train, we do not train at the expense of the normal lives we live.

When Normal People find something we love to do, we do not usually want to do it only once or even just for a just short while; we want to keep doing it for as long as we can. While I came to ultrarunning comparatively late at forty-six years old, I knew it was something I wanted to keep doing. But I also knew that it was something I wanted to keep being able to do.

What this means for Normal People, at least for those of us who fall in love with ultrarunning, is that to stay with the sport beyond our first race, we must prepare not only for the race but also for the day after we cross that first finish line.

We must put a life training plan into place, one that is separate from, independent of, and in addition to any race training plan we may choose to tackle. A life training plan is one that lies beneath everything we do. It is about maintaining focus on our everyday lives—the foundation we create and maintain, even the mundane aspects. When a Normal Person takes on a life training plan, it ensures a high level of daily health and happiness—high enough to make not only our next race possible but also the next after that.

Training for daily health and happiness is much harder than training for an ultramarathon. It takes more focus, more consistency, and more discipline. Life training is ongoing and does not end until we end. Life training takes great attention and awareness. Ultramarathon training has a tangible goal sitting out there in the future and a clear endgame. To always be in training requires an ongoing decision to never allow ourselves to be swept away by anything that turns us off to the quality of our normal lives. Normal people need breaks, but we cannot afford to take significant time off. In a successful life, there are no on and off "seasons" of training. Successful Normal People are always on.

Adopting an always-in-training mindset has massive payoffs. It is a mindset of taking the long view, understanding that our actions are not about getting through the day but rather succeeding in our lives. We become hyperaware of when our stress is becoming too great or not great enough, then we adjust as needed. We make the adjustments because we want to continue living good lives. In this way, we can continue doing what we love without burning out or stagnating. With an always-in-training mindset, we are laser focused on always improving ourselves, on building and maintaining a strong platform of existence off which to jump and on which to land.

While there is definitely something incredible about the over-sixty-year-olds and over-seventy-year-olds who finish my race each year, it is not magic. There are explainable factors and reasons for their success that exist well outside of genetics. I believe that if we were to delve into the particulars of their lives, we would recognize some themes much in the way we see through lines in the world's so-called "Blue Zones," small pockets of people around the world who are the healthiest and live the longest. While these communities live in different parts of the world, they share the following: predominantly plant-based diets, moderate alcohol consumption, daily but not significantly stressful movement, multigenerational family members in the community or under the same roof, positive mindsets, and a connection to nature. With some perspective, it is easy to see that humans who eat well, live lives with true social connection, engage in joyful and healthy activities, and cope with managed stress do the business of life better than those who do not. They live better and longer overall.

A Normal Person who is always in training will similarly live better and longer overall. Though the picture might look different from one Normal Person to another, the following factors are vital to a healthy, balanced life.

Exercise: The Normal Person exercises most days but not in a particularly stressful way: light jogs, walks, swims, bikes, some strength training, often half an hour to an hour, five or six days per week. Normal People take days off when needed. If and when we feel fatigued, we have not been sleeping well, or we are otherwise under-resourced, Normal People prioritize what we need to get back on track over hitting data points or completing training regimens. Normal People may seek assistance or inspiration from others or from tools—such as step counting—to help us move throughout our days. Ensuring that these tools inspire us to move in ways that provides energy rather than depleting us of it (i.e., by overtraining) is vital.

Diet: Normal People eat healthy food most days but do not overly manage food choices or intake too much, especially when out with friends, at parties, or traveling. Similar to how Normal People relate to exercise, eating well is not about micromanaging diet, counting calories, or any other such method of unnecessary control. Normal People eat well most of the time and adjust as needed when fatigued, depleted of energy, or when becoming under- or overweight. Because we are always in training, these adjustments are not wide swings, crash diets, or seven-day cleanses. They require just a bit of attention applied to eating habits—periodically minor course corrections.

Breathwork: Normal People do the hard work of stress management in the way we eat and move but also in modalities such as breathwork and meditation. Normal People, in general, are busy with work and family and thus don't prioritize spending forty-five minutes sitting in front of a candle every day. We develop a habit of active awareness through meditation and attention to breath in the middle of our lives. During exercise, meals, work, and socializing, Normal People work hard to be present.

Sleep: Normal People, always in training, place a high value on sleep quality. We keep a relatively regular sleep schedule most days, spending some time winding down at the end of each day. We keep caffeine, alcohol, and marijuana intake managed and minimized. A good night's sleep has as much to do with the quality (i.e., the amount of deep sleep) as the quantity. Caffeine, alcohol, marijuana, sleeping pills, and other drugs can disrupt the quality of sleep, even though we may be asleep for the same amount of hours.

Socialization: Normal People work to establish a healthy balance of socializing and solitude. When it comes to spending time with friends and family, we value quality over quantity. We limit social media, and we are keenly aware of the negative implications of spending too much time or energy engaging with it. We make time for socializing, but we have the strength to say no when we need or want to.

Please refer to the Resources section (page 141) for more detail on these factors.

Though the factors above are important considerations for leading healthier, happier lives, "always being in training" is a mindset. It is a mindset that values the whole, the bigger picture, and refrains from measuring one's life by a win or loss on any particular day. For example, I often help clients see that healthy eating is never about a single meal but rather about the totality of one's diet—how we eat most of the time. (I call it their "MOTT.") These clients may have lost a single battle around food, perhaps by overeating or binging, but they often fail to recognize that most of the time they are eating quite well and better than ever before. Always being in training awards us the ability and perspective to notice the overall trajectory of our lives in lieu of beating ourselves up over single events or even single days. By adopting this mindset, we come to understand that success exists in patterns, not one-offs. The always-in-training Normal Person is prepared for the multiple battles and struggles inherent in a good, long, healthy life—a life that Normal People want.

Normal People do not *want* to burn out. We do not *want* to push ourselves to the point of injury. We do not *want* to act in ways that keep us from the normal lives we want to live. Yet without specific tools in place and a proper mindset to help avoid these actions, burn out we will and burn out we often do. We will push ourselves too hard without even being aware we are doing so. If we were elite athletes, we would push harder and harder and go for the win. When Normal People engage life in this way, we act in conflict with our larger, profoundly more important goal of a good life. While training only for a race, we ignore how training for everything else that makes up our non-race lives makes all the difference.

I embarked on the adventure of running ultramarathons and found in it something I wanted to keep doing. This meant that

I had to come to the same realization that many Normal People who fall in love with trail ultrarunning do: in order to continue with this out-of-the-box act, we must attend to what is happening "inside of the box."

Ultrarunning teaches Normal People
to always be in training.

To Go from Aid Station to Aid Station

> Great things are not done by impulse, but by a series of things brought together.

— VINCENT VAN GOGH

I toed the line of the fifty-miler in the worst possible head-space: waking up in the dark, early hours of the morning; riding a flimsy school bus to the starting line; lying on cold, unforgiving asphalt seemingly for hours as fatigue settled into my bones and I questioned everything related to why I was there; listening for the starting gun in a sea of people—all of these factors had built heavily on each other, and I wished I were just about anywhere else. I stood there thinking, "This is the last place I want to be right now." Not a promising beginning for anyone about to run most of the day—eleven hours and fifty-two minutes, to be precise—over some pretty rough terrain and an extreme distance.

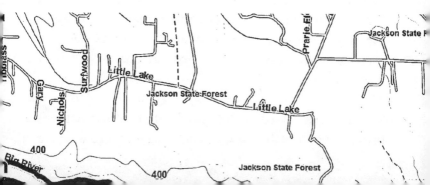

What followed was certainly not the result of a preconceived game plan, some strategy that I had penned in a notebook along with a specific nutrition plan and finish-time goal. Instead, what followed was an on-the-fly strategy of necessity and one without which I very likely would have turned right around, cabbed it back to the hotel, and climbed back into a comfy, warm hotel bed with my wife. This strategy, which I repeated to myself throughout the race, was "I'll just run to the next aid station and see how I feel."

That was what got me not just to the starting line but over it. I pushed the reality of the fifty miles out of my head and replaced it with a brand-new, manageable goal that took off some of the pressure: "I'll just run to the first aid station and see how I feel." And off I ran.

When I arrived at the first aid station, about five miles in, my stomach was indeed a little wonky. I felt some light nausea and general discomfort. It was very early in the morning, and I was still warming up, so I knew that I was not in too bad of shape. My mood had even improved slightly. The sun had come up, seemingly erasing both the morning's cold darkness and my rather sour mood. I took a short break of a few minutes at the aid station, topped off my bottles, put my pack back on, and headed back out. Again, I thought, "I'll just run to the next aid station and see how I feel." Even this early in the race, the finish line had all but vanished from my field of concern. It had become some faint idea so far in the future that it was not worth significant thought or consideration. My only reality and my sole challenge were getting to the next aid station. This narrow field of focus kept me moving.

This approach worked extremely well at the race start, but even better at the inevitable I-want-to-quit stage of the race I wrote about earlier. My wife met me at the mile-twenty-nine aid station, and despite the nausea and general stomach discomfort having largely subsided, the fatigue and strain had begun to really settle in. Running twenty-nine miles might normally be seen as something to feel good about, and in isolation, it would be. But the awareness that I was still looking at twenty-one more miles kept me in such a low place. I predicted, unfortunately correctly, that I would be facing another rough patch ahead. But my wife had done some of her own course research and discovered an optimal meeting location at mile forty. Later, I marveled at how odd the human brain is because, to me in this fatigued state, mile forty was *only eleven more miles*. Compared to the finish line twenty-one miles away, the eleven seemed to be—incredibly—not that big of a deal. "I'll see her again at mile forty, I'll see her again at mile forty, I'll see her again at mile forty," I repeated to myself. Interestingly, the fact that the forty-mile mark was a mere ten miles from the finish did not even occur to me at the time. Even being that much closer to the finish line, my mindset was still squarely settled in just getting to the next aid station. And it was working.

My wife recorded me coming in at mile forty for the YouTube video I later made recounting the race. In the footage, I look absolutely floored. At that point in the race, I had just completed a particularly brutal ten-mile stretch of constant ups and downs with almost zero flats. It was not only physically draining but mentally as well, and it showed. I walked up to her, sat on a metal railing, and offered an exasperated report of what had just occurred. I hung out with her for a few minutes, telling her that I had no idea whether I'd encounter any more of that insane terrain.

While I could have intricately researched the course prior to race day and familiarized myself with what was to come, my approach has always been to eschew this kind of knowledge, even more so after all that I'd learned from my race experiment. On one hand, I would not have been confronted with the surprise craziness of so much climbing, but on the other, knowing about the craziness ahead of time would have been stress-inducing—and long before race day. I had trained for a hard race no matter what, and the extra stress leading up to race day wouldn't have helped anything. I am, after all, a Normal Person, and that stress would have detracted from all the other areas of my Normal Person's life.

My very favorite part of the video occurs as I leave my wife to embark on the final ten miles of the race. As I head toward the trail, a stranger, keenly aware of my intense level of fatigue, exclaims, "You've got this, man!" Without the energy to even turn around to face him, I throw up a half-hearted wave, and off I go. Looking back at the video, I take pride in that moment: to quit then and there would have been so, so easy and certainly more comfortable. But off I went because, in my mind, what lay before me was just another fairly manageable segment of distance, just another point in the near future toward which to head.

Crossing that finish line felt otherworldly. My eldest daughter joined me for the last fifty feet of the fifty-mile beast, and to this day, it is the part of the race I remember and cherish most. The physical and mental highs were palpable. As proof that ultrarunning, like other endurance sports, is mostly a mental feat, I was able to run the last part of the race quite well, even though several miles prior I had felt as though I could barely even walk. In any case, that day's strategy of going from one aid station to the next enabled me to win the day, enabled me to *feel* the finish. It's the strategy that delivered me the experience that I still keep in my back pocket and bring with me to every race since that first fifty-miler.

Watching the video, I can see my fatigue. Rationally, I know it was there that day, but I cannot still feel it. We humans have an odd but useful ability to block out or entirely forget struggles and pain once we are past them. We know they were there. We remember the details of the painful event—the location, the weather, other people, the time. We *know* we got our asses kicked, but we cannot quite fully relive that part of it. We cannot refeel the misery. The high we feel after such an experience, like crossing an ultramarathon finish line, effectively diminishes most of the memory of pain.

> *After completing an ultramarathon, Normal People often experience for the first time a knowledge that we are capable of so much more than we previously thought possible. And this knowledge feels so good that we intentionally and consciously invite the experience again in spite of the fact that we rationally know it will bring us more pain. We welcome it for that intense feeling of being alive.*

Through facing my own challenges and helping others face theirs, I have come to recognize what I believe is a psychological throughline in our species: when faced with what we perceive to be an enormously huge goal, we are easily stopped in our tracks. But I have also come to recognize a second throughline: we can accomplish that same goal when we break it down into smaller, more manageable chunks that we then meet one at a time on our way to the literal or figurative finish line.

I built my entire Small Steps coaching practice on this concept. By empowering my clients with the ability to break up their lofty and noble goals of better health and happiness into small steps, they are able not only to reach their goals but also to keep them. Importantly, the size of each "small" step is relative to the client and their life, motivation, and baseline level of stress. Without this strategy, the best most of us can do is to ride the short-term excitement that the mere idea of the big goal elicits: "I'm going to lose fifty pounds in thirty days!" or "I'm going to meditate for one hour every day starting tomorrow!" or "Once I get a better job, I'm going to hit the gym for an hour a day!" We ride this wave of excitement only for a short period of time before inevitably quitting just as soon as the excitement wanes, and then we are faced with the reality of the actual hard work that awaits us. This reality has led to the popularity of the ever soul-crushing quick-fix diets and fitness plans.

Small Stepping is a mindset in and of itself, looking at our lives from a backdrop of what I call the "ethic of self-care." We may learn about something we want to take on (e.g., how to eat healthier, exercise, meditate, paint, etc.) but ultimately our success depends on how we implement that knowledge. In other words, it is less about what we know and more about how well we take care of ourselves in the process of applying that knowledge to our lives. Excitement aside, diets are tough—we make initial gains and feel wonderful about ourselves, but then ... because we took on too much too soon, we cannot sustain it, and not only does the weight come back but we feel like we have failed. As I tell my clients, time is our only enemy—the question is whether we can manage our stress well enough during the implementation process such that we stick with any new behavior long enough for it to become a habit. Regardless of how much we may know, can we begin with a manageable, smaller action and then build from there?

My Small Steps approach dovetailed seamlessly with my foray into trail ultrarunning. Living as a "Small Stepper" and running a trail ultramarathon are both first and foremost about stress management. Both are about keeping a keen eye on avoiding overwhelm and burnout. Both are about setting up interim benchmarks that we perceive as achievable without an inordinate amount of stress. Both are about playing the long game—not doing too much too soon to prevent quitting before reaching the finish line. In my Small Stepping world, the finish line is any desired behavior becoming an actual habit. In an ultramarathon, the finish line is, well ... the finish line.

What stops Normal People from attempting an ultramarathon, and thus the otherworldly feeling of crossing the finish line, is that we cannot even fathom the idea in the first place. It sounds just *too* crazy. But when we do make the decision to go for it, we substantially increase our chances of finishing by breaking up the race, and even our training, into smaller goals along the way—aid station to aid station. Soon enough, Normal People come to recognize the enormous benefit of applying this strategy and mindset to each and every big goal we have—writing a book, going back to school, or learning an instrument. This aid-station-to-aid-station mindset gets us moving toward our goals precisely at the moment we set them. We realize there is a way to reach mountaintops that most others will not even attempt to climb—by mapping out and tackling shorter, seemingly manageable climbs along the way until we find ourselves at the peak.

*Ultrarunning teaches Normal People to
go from aid station to aid station.*

To See That We Are All in This Together

We are like islands in the sea, separate on the surface but connected in the deep.

— WILLIAM JAMES

A large part of my effort to share the benefits of ultrarunning with Normal People is based on my personal experience. I never took to road races, but trail running became my passion. I know plenty of people who do not enjoy running on trails, and certainly not for the "crazy" ultra-distances. However, the draw of trail ultrarunning's *ultra* aspect is just as important as the *trail* aspect. In other words, it is both the trails *and* being on them for a good long while that hold tremendous value for any Normal Person stepping into the trail-ultrarunning world. It's the entire ultrarunning package that delivers a life-changing experience for Normal People. If we can move through our fear, question the assumptions and perceptions we have about ourselves, and finally come to understand that failure is solely not trying in the first place, we Normal People can give ultramarathoning a

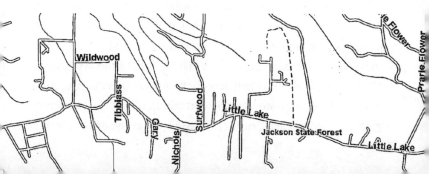

shot. When we do, we become part of a relatively small group of people who have firsthand experience with this very under-the-radar event.

At the core of my desire for more Normal People to become trail ultrarunners is the knowledge that this sport has the capacity to break us down in a way that perhaps no other sport can. It puts us in a raw state, a wonderfully raw state. And when we are there, a truth finds its way to the surface. A truth that is often shoved down and kept down by social media and the news: an understanding that we all have much more in common than we think. Whatever pretense, arrogance, overconfidence, anger, keyboard bravado, machismo, stubbornness, or intolerance that we wear into the world is stripped from us when we are left raw. We simply do not have the energy for any of it. What we are left with in this state is empathy, vulnerability, kindness, com-passion, and presence. Perhaps surprising to some, all Normal People possess all of these characteristics.

Races are social for Normal People. We do not show up to win the race, and while some of us may shoot for a personal best, we appreciate and even crave the comradery, the shared expe-rience, often above the competitive aspect. If it were *just* about completing a fixed distance or setting a personal record, we might just as easily go out solo on any random day, but we do not. We crave the adrenaline of race day, which often comes from being with and around all the other runners. There is a tribal element to races, and we are both connected to it and by it. We feel the energy that compounds when we are in the presence of so many other nervous runners. And it feels good to be part of a shared experience. The nature of these physical challenges breaks us down, which inspires in us a deep-seated desire to look out for everyone with whom we are experiencing it. In my hardest races, runners have always come up beside me to make sure I was doing okay. These kinds of interactions are not anomalies. I have heard stories of professional ultrarunners helping their competitors stay on the course when clearly *not* doing so would've ensured an advantage at the finish line.

Prior to my first ultramarathon, I had run half-marathons, marathons, 10Ks, and even the Spartan Race. Each was challenging—especially the Spartan Race, which was definitely one of the most difficult things I have ever done and why I will forever loathe tractor tires—and each has its own special attributes and character. People love them and participate in them for various reasons. But none of these events is an ultramarathon, and none of them contains the raw potential for true growth and change that ultramarathons possess. For one thing, ultras are still fairly unknown. Everyone has heard of marathons and half-marathons, and most have heard of obstacle races, but very few are familiar with ultramarathons—or the fact that they take place on trails. The big question is inevitably "What makes a race an ultramarathon?" People are rather shocked when they find out. "Wait . . . it's longer than 26.2 miles?" they ask incredulously. And they're even more shocked when they hear the details: the trails, streams, rocks, roots, and steep ascents and descents. Perhaps because the sport is a mystery to most Normal People, ultramarathons have an aura about them that the more mainstream events do not.

This aura means that when Normal People toe the line of an ultramarathon, we are going be hyperaware of the crazy thing we are choosing to do, and this realization is shared by all the other Normal People surrounding us who *also* think that what they themselves are about to embark upon is crazy. This common reality fosters an empathy and facilitates a connection among the runners. While it never feels good to be afraid, it feels a whole hell of a lot better to be afraid with others who are either just as afraid as we are or were *this* afraid at some point in their past, as in at the starting line of their first ultramarathon attempt. During these moments, no competition with "the other" exists. What exists in its place is a let's-get-through-this-together mentality.

In my experience, this level of togetherness does not occur nearly as much in the rah-rah nature of the bigger, more corporate, adrenaline-junkie events like the Spartan Race. There is some serious physical breakdown during these events to be sure, but of a louder, different nature than what occurs during an ultramarathon, where any breakdown is met with quieter support, fewer spectators, less fanfare, and longer hours.

The first of the only two marathons I have ever run, the CIM in Sacramento, was supposedly a good first marathon—the course was relatively flat and the race took place during winter, away from the hottest months. I got through the race fine, but a couple things stood out to me apart from the misery of a bus ride to the starting line at four-thirty in the morning. The first was the sheer number of runners—over ten thousand (compared to the one hundred fifty runners who participate each year in the ultra I direct). The second was a series of signs with various times noted on them, held by runners at the starting line. Initially puzzled, I quickly realized what these were: if a runner had a specific finish-time goal in mind, they could run next to the corresponding sign for that pace during the race to help them cross the finish line at their desired time. So if someone was looking to run a nine-minute mile, they would find the volunteer runner holding the nine-minute sign and run with them during the race.

Once ultrarunners hit a single-track trail, it is impossible to run in groups, much less next to a person holding a sign—and given the terrain, even holding a sign in the first place would be a feat in and of itself, and quite dangerous. Substantive conversations between runners are a challenge when running single file. As a result, runners settle into quiet, as attention to terrain becomes a priority and necessity. The limited social interaction is taxing. On remote trails, runners cannot even rely on the support of spectators. Ultramarathon courses are rarely lined with people cheering and offering messages and signs of energetic support. Ultrarunners get some support from enthusiastic and highly appreciated aid station volunteers, but, like the aid stations themselves, these volunteers are few and far between. The solo in-your-own-head-for-a-really-long-time experience is part of what peels away so much of all the distractions the outside world has to offer. But with less conversation—or perhaps because of it—we feel that we are really *with* the other runners, sharing an unspoken struggle, a presence, and a vulnerability. Everyone is in their own heads yet all together.

In ultramarathons, we are traveling to a destination to be sure—the finish line—but the sheer distance, time, silence, and solitude allow us to get lost in moments along the way, to periodically forget about the finish line. In a sense, we are liberated from constantly looking forward, and we have moments when we find ourselves with nothing to do except look at and listen to what is around us. From time to time, we might hear the breathing and footsteps of a fellow runner as they pass us or we pass them, and with that, a quick hello or a brief and pleasant exchange. There is no discussion of politics, and there are no questions of religion, only an uncommon depth of shared experience.

In these moments, we connect to a mutual feeling and an unspoken acknowledgment: "I bet you feel as bad as I do, and there is comfort in that for both of us."

How valuable and how increasingly rare these times are in our lives—times when we find connection with people with whom we almost surely would've assumed there to be none. And what a stark contrast between these connections and those on social media—where they're not so much "connections" as interactions that never get to the core of who we are as humans. Interactions that never get deep enough to unearth the challenges we all are going through or the desire we all have to get through this life the best we can for as long as we can.

And there, amid all the noise of the world, is trail ultrarunning. There, in the shadows of the "not yet mainstream," ultrarunning continues to bring more and more Normal People into the fold and, in its relative smallness, offers us a protection from both external and comparative pressures. The act of ultrarunning, at least for now, is inherently personal and largely private. But precisely because it is so, it foments a very real connection between human beings. During an ultramarathon, in moments of rarely otherwise experienced fatigue and pain, we find strength in both giving and receiving encouragement. We understand on a fundamental level that the humans around us are feeling what we are feeling, questioning what we are questioning, and fearing what we are fearing. There is a true comfort in that knowledge and then, rising up from inside of us, a true desire to make things better for everyone around us, not *just* for ourselves.

Ultrarunning teaches Normal People
that we are all in this together.

To Test Our Mettle

> To dare is to lose one's footing momentarily. Not to dare is to lose oneself.

— SØREN KIERKEGAARD

Some Normal People who run my ultramarathon cross the finish line in tears.

I cap my registration list at no more than one hundred fifty participants, and doing so enables me to greet every single runner as they cross the finish line. This is a point of pride for me as it embodies yet another aspect of the truly personal nature of the sport. Finishers exhibit a wide range of emotions—pure fatigue, pure joy, pure relief, pure pride—sometimes all at the same time, and often this surge of emotion manifests in tears. But the word that best describes the state of a Normal Person crossing the finish line of a trail ultramarathon is "raw."

The raw tears that running an ultramarathon inspire are a special brand of tears. They are not just tears of joy, nor just tears

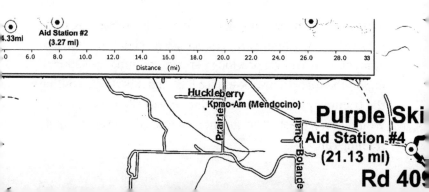

of sadness, though joy and sadness are certainly wrapped up in them. They are tears of a sacrifice of time and sleep, a defiance of expectations, and an achievement of a crazy goal. Embodied in every ultramarathoner's finish is the culmination of worry, fear, strife, dedication, sacrifice, commitment, and hard work—so much hard work, so much shifting of schedules to get a run in, so many early mornings, so much at stake, so much self-imposed pressure. Crossing the finish line makes the unknown known. Given all of this, it actually surprises me that not all runners cry.

The self-imposed pressure and expectations are intense. We arrive on race day believing that all our training will mean nothing if we are unable to finish. We think all our work will be for naught. During the many hours on the trails, our minds drift in and out of self-doubt, confrontation with a perceived impossibility, and fear of what people will think if we do not finish (the same people who thought we were crazy for even trying, and who will most certainly feel validated if we do not succeed, but succeed by their measure of success, not ours). Yet, at the same time, when Normal People do finish an ultramarathon, we might wonder: If this is possible, what else is possible? What if we can achieve even more, substantially more, than we think we can? By crossing that finish line for the first time, action disproves our perceptions, reality disproves our expectations—it is no longer about what we believed we could achieve but what we actually have achieved.

I vividly remember training for my first ultra: learning to be versatile in my training, experiencing a level of attention and awareness I had never previously known, learning the supreme importance of breathwork and the like. And this was just during the training phase. But above all that was the big unknown: Would I even finish? The question haunted me on every single training run.

One of my favorite runs to this day is along the Big River, about a fifteen-minute drive from my house and right across from the Stanford Inn & Resort. The path stretches for miles along the river. In fact, the first ten miles of the race I direct goes mostly along this path before cutting off into some serious hills and single-track trails. I frequented this path during the early days of my training. At that point, I was quite unfamiliar with the local trails and tended to get lost, but the Big River trail was an out-and-back with virtually no easy way to get lost. Depending on the miles I was assigned on a given day, I would run in for the first half, then back out for the second half. After the first five or so runs, a spot on the trail about three and a half miles in became my pretend finish line. I would run a ten-miler and upon hitting the five-mile mark, I would turn around and head back, and there it would be—this particular section about three and a half miles from the starting point. What drew me to it was one interesting and relevant feature: a tree that at some point had lain across the path but that had since been removed. What remained was a fairly distinct line of shredded wood and dust. In my mind, that line was a finish line. The finish line.

I would "see" people standing there, I'd "hear" loud music, and I'd picture myself running across the line. It did not matter that I had no idea what the actual finish line would be like. What mattered was that I was doing the work to get my mind in the place of finishing. I was trying, regardless of how futile, to know an unknown, to grab any bit of confidence and familiarity I could. This became a regular practice and one that I began to look forward to every time I ran on that particular trail. Now, six years later, when I run past that same point from time to time, I'm transported immediately back to that intense state of apprehension, anxiety, fear, and unknowing. It is a fond memory ... What we do not know in general can be frightening, but being faced with something specific about ourselves (for instance, whether we will finish an ultramarathon) can be paralyzing. So paralyzing, in fact, that for many Normal People, this not knowing is more than enough to keep us from even trying.

So why try, then? What truly is the point of these self-administered searches of our limits? Is this just some sort of adrenaline-junkie act, some act of insecurity that we think will prove to the world how tough we are? Is there any real, personal value in pushing ourselves? Can pushing ourselves from time to time lead us to discover what we are capable of, especially in light of everything in today's world that makes it so easy to not push ourselves?

I do believe there is real value in testing our limits, and stepping far outside our comfort zones every now and then might be the most valuable act a Normal Person can do. There are several reasons that I believe this to be true.

The first reason is relativity. When we push ourselves and discover what we are capable of, momentarily touching on an extreme in the process, our so-called "regular" problems and "regular" lives become relatively less stressful. A big push elicits a built-in, automatic influx of perspective, and suddenly the mundane ceases to carry as much weight as it previously did. The week after an ultramarathon, a stressful incident at work or a tiff with a spouse suddenly seems relatively unimportant. After all, compared to a 50K trail run, office drama is small change.

The second reason is awareness. In pushing ourselves into periods of inordinate effort, we come to greater appreciate the things that matter most to us but from which we are otherwise easily distracted—all that often goes underappreciated or unnoticed in the busyness and craziness of our Normal People lives. Temporary big pushes transport us to a deeper existence with a renewed and refreshed attention to what is truly important. In essence, any step outside of our routines wakes us up and shakes us up. We even come to notice the routines themselves and either take comfort in them or realize we need to change them. The job to which we have been going day in and day out begins to look just a little different. We take a different route to work or notice a shop we had not noticed before. A big push is a figurative kick in the pants reminding us of what is important and what makes us truly happy.

I live in a beautiful area. The Mendocino coast of California is ripe with fields, redwood forests, and rivers, and its rugged bluffs touch the Pacific Ocean. Registering for that first ultramarathon took me to the trails, to places that inspire me to recognize and appreciate where I live. Virtually every day I notice the trees and the ocean on the way to work. I appreciate the lack of traffic and congestion, and I appreciate having left both behind in Los Angeles. I feel a greater perspective in both my work life and family life. Of course, there are stressful days, but fewer and further between, and I seem to be able to recover and move on more quickly from them.

While I would never attribute this shift in my life solely to running ultramarathons, I can say that the races are ever present in my mind. Those experiences taught me the ability to better assess what is happening, and I find that, in most cases, what is happening simply is not as important or as challenging as I might have previously thought, especially in the grander scheme of things. Ultrarunning has played an important role in my being able to see the big picture and avoid being swept up in what, on some level, I know I do not truly care about.

The third reason is confidence. There exist a strength and confidence in the mere attempt at something great. The litany of inspirational quotes trying to convince everyone of the necessity of failure in order to succeed may be the most easier-said-than-done advice for a successful life, but this does not make them any less true. Failing, especially when devoid of perspective, feels horrible and can easily prevent Normal People from ever attempting anything bold.

But in making the intentional choice even just to see what we might be able do, to take a shot at hitting our limits, we come to realize a very profound truth: a successful life lies in the search itself.

We must be willing to succeed. With this mindset in place, the finish line begins to lose its luster just as the starting line gains brightness. Although this fact never fully erases the disappointment of not finishing a race, it hones our minds to an awareness that we are stronger Normal People for toeing the line in the first place. In doing so, we widen the divide between those who dare and those who are afraid to dare. We gain confidence by the mere act of showing up. And we will keep showing up.

Aspiring for greatness is no easy task when it is all too easy to lower our own expectations for ourselves. There is safety and comfort when we lower the bar on our lives, and this explains why the world is filled to the brim with people living this reality—living but not feeling alive. For, on some level, it is technically true that if we do not attempt the challenge in the first place, we cannot fail at it. But as the clichés tell us, we cannot succeed either, especially when we see that true success is about the big picture of a happy life. A life that is always much bigger than a finish line.

Just registering for my first ultramarathon triggered an immediate what-have-I-done? elevated heart rate and a why-am-I-doing-this? shortness of breath. Just the act of clicking the payment button revved up my mental engine. All the worries in my mind momentarily heightened. And then, I thought, "How odd a species we are." Here I was, choosing to click the button. In that moment of elevated stress and anxiety, I had both the power and the ability to change my mind and cancel the registration or, even easier, to have chosen not to register in the first place. Yet I clicked the button just the same. In that moment, my training began.

I believe that most Normal People can (and should) run an ultramarathon. Even writing that sentence feels odd, even though I write it as a Normal Person who has completed multiple ultramarathons. I can picture readers still thinking how crazy an idea it is, how completely outside the realm of possibility running an ultramarathon *feels* for most people. While this may be true, these are, in fact, only feelings. Most people *feel* they could never do it, *feel* it is insane, *feel* it is just not them. But remember that nobody actually *knows* until they attempt it. We must acknowledge that all too often, our feelings do not align with facts. It is a position of strength to question our feelings from time to time, to ask whether what we feel matches up with what we know or do not know—about ourselves and about the world. Ultramarathons elicit strong feelings to be sure, but to understand that we do not and cannot really know whether we'll finish means we can move those feelings to the side and press on. So often it is fulfilling and enlivening to proceed with what we know *in spite of* what we feel—to move through fear—and when we do, we are stronger for it.

I believe most Normal People can (and should) run an ultramarathon, precisely because most of us believe it to be a crazy thing to do. Over time, this adventurous, testing-the-waters mindset bleeds into our Normal Person lives just as every other lesson in this book does.

To put ourselves out there. To test our limits. To step outside the norm. To take the fight to our lives. To break up our routines. To be versatile. To feel connected. To breathe. To improve ourselves. To question our feelings. To feel alive. To stretch our minds. To find our true character. To move through fear. To confront failure. To define success.

Ultrarunning teaches Normal People to test our mettle.

Epilogue

All the Lessons Again

As I write this, I am in the process of wrapping up the sixth year of the Mendocino Coast 50K, the race I created and direct. It was another incredible year. Runners from over fifteen states in the US and from South Africa, Japan, and Canada descended upon my small town for a breathtaking thirty-two-mile loop of the Big River, redwoods, creeks, waterfalls, and technical trails, leading finally to the cliffs touching the edge of the Pacific.

Putting on this race takes an incredible amount of work, including from the fantastic and supremely crucial volunteers that make the actual day happen. But all the work leading up to race day is handled by a skeleton crew: my friend Brie, the assistant race director; me, during the months prior; then my wife (and sometimes even my children) and Cyd during the last few days. This race is truly a labor of love, and while each year there are inevitably more than a few moments when I swear this will be the last time that I do this, as soon as I greet the first runners across the finish line, I know I will be back.

One of my favorite parts is the day before the race each year, when my good friend Skip Brand (founder of Healdsburg Running Company and writer of this book's foreword) and I run the course, checking the trails and course markings (competently done in advance by a local cycling club) and adding some additional marking tape of our own. Cyd is our "crew" for the day, meeting us at three locations along the course with fruit, water, coconut water, ginger chews (a favorite of mine on long runs), and a welcomed break. Running the day before the race gives me the unique ability to deliver a thorough report to the runners: what to look out for on the trails, how deep the river crossing is, and other pertinent information. For many first-time ultramarathoners, of which my race attracts a fair amount, this report is a bit of a confidence boost, as is the fact that I am up and about, having finished the course only some hours before.

Skip and I have run this every year, and I cherish the tradition. But this year's run took on an unexpected and special meaning for me—so much so, in fact, that I was inspired to write this epilogue:

As the race date approaches, my stress proportionally increases. About four months before the figurative starting gun fires (I usually just say "Go!"), I begin wading through hundreds of to-dos: renting the supply truck; ordering reusable silicon cups, hoodies, hats, etched "finisher" beer glasses, or other swag I land on each year; plus coordinating catering and much, much more. Two days before race day, my wife and I organize the aid station supplies and pack up the supply truck, including thirty five-gallon jugs of water. This process involves significant physical work, and throughout the day, one thought rises in my mind above all the others: "Tomorrow I will be running a thirty-two-mile trail ultramarathon." I feel fear and dread, anxiety and stress. I am super busy and physically active loading a supply truck, but I *should* be resting; I *should* be taking the day off. And then, yet another thought emerges: "The day *after* I run the thirty-two miles on trails is race day. Race day . . . when I will be getting up at 4:00 a.m., driving the supply truck to the start/finish, and engaging in even more physical work by setting up the tables, chairs, and road signs. I'll be on my feet all day, greeting the runners before and after the race and dealing with all the inevitable unknowns. So many unknowns. More anxiety, more stress. More physical work . . ."

That is how it has been and how it was again this year.

This year, it was all the same stuff except for one significant difference: this book, full of all the lessons ultrarunning has taught me, concretized into these pages. Each lesson was fresh and present in my mind before, during, and after the race. So fresh, in fact, that only five days prior to my running the course with Skip, I had turned in the most recent draft to my editor and publisher. So fresh that, in the days leading up to running the course as well as the race day itself, I had the odd experience not of only feeling everything I wrote about in the book but also noticing the fact that I was feeling it all, that keen self-awareness.

In a sense, I was watching this book play out in real time. "I just need to get to the next location where Cyd is meeting us, and, oh, right, this is the part of the book where I wrote about learning the value of running from aid station to aid station." This book could have been the narrator for the week of the race. My years of experience delivered me the confidence to write this book in the first place, but reexperiencing it all, with the learned lessons and internalized truths already distilled on the page, instilled in me an additional confidence that other Normal People might learn from this sport what I have learned.

To move through fear:

The fear of not getting enough sleep the night before running, even though I knew I would not and never have before any previous race. The fear that I would not finish the course or that

I might get injured. The fear was present, and it was real. Yet I made no effort to make it go away, and by not doing so, I had a great day with friends on the course.

To slow down:

As expected, starting out with Skip, I felt like running a bit quicker than usual. The excitement of the day and my nervous energy and anxiety were clearly afoot. But within the first one hundred yards, I said to Skip, "I need to take it easy." I made the effort to slow down, and in doing so, I made the day a great success—much better, in fact, than the previous year.

To be versatile:

By most running-book training-plan standards, I was severely undertrained, but as I crested mile thirty-two, I was so thankful that the inclusion of breathwork, a healthy diet, and strength training to my overall training regimen paid off extremely well.

To pay attention in everything:

More than ever before, I stole moments on the course and appreciated the natural beauty: the trails, trees, waterfalls, river, and ocean. I was also more present on the trails with Skip and more involved at the makeshift aid stations with Cyd and Cyd's boyfriend, Adam, this year. I appreciated this yearly tradition in a way I had not in years past.

To breathe:

The nasal-only breathing, employed all throughout the course except during extreme inclines, was indispensable. My attention to breath enabled me to effectively manage my stress and regulate my pace. I remained mostly calm, aware, and present. I listened to my breath and paid attention to my ability (or inability) to keep it regulated.

To always be in training:

As you've found out by now, I am not a natural athlete nor a great one, and given the relatively minimal miles I run on a typical week (about ten to twelve, mostly on a treadmill), most would balk at the idea that I would ever have been able to complete the thirty-two miles in the first place, much less to continue with the physical demands of the prerace prep, race-day duties, and postrace cleanup, then return to my regular job at the resort the following day. But I take care of myself most of the time. I strive to always be in training—my MOTT (most of the time) efforts are focused on stress management and all the factors that point to it and affect it: a healthy diet, varied exercise, quality sleep, cold therapy, breathwork, and periodic breaks and days off. All of these factors have become normal, regular aspects of my life, and each contributes to a strong foundation of health and happiness that enables me to hit some periodic larger challenges.

To go from aid station to aid station:

Even though the thirty-two-mile run with Skip was not an organized race with aid stations, we still followed this approach to running the course. Cyd and Adam met us at three locations we'd agreed on ahead of time. Cyd, a seasoned ultramarathoner in her own right, has an eerie ability to fairly accurately predict our arrival time to each location—not an easy feat with so much variation in the terrain. In my mind, these locations were the aid stations, and I used them as I would during an official race: to break down the large, overall (stress-inducing) distance into mentally manageable chunks, with the thought "I just gotta get to the next aid station." That approach made the day flow well, and I avoided the gargantuan-goal paralysis that likely would have occurred if I had expended any mental energy focusing on the total number of miles I had to cover that day.

To see that we are all in this together:

The race-day experience, even with the seemingly unavoidable hiccups, far outweighed all the stress and hard work leading up to it. Supported by the intimate nature of a race capped at one hundred fifty registrants, I appreciated being able to personally greet every runner as they crossed the finish line. And as with the previous races, tears, relief, and joy abounded. The emotional answer to the question in every Normal Person's mind at the beginning of the race: Can I do this?

I counted down to the start, and about seven to eight hours later, most runners came in and were hanging out, eating, and socializing. This is another part of the day I treasure—clearly witnessing the fact that there is little if any separation between all of us, economics, race, religion, politics, gender, and age barriers having melted away. We are humans sharing a common experience. We are connected by a common effort. All of us are connected.

To test our mettle:

I was dreading the thirty-two miles. I felt pressure, albeit self-imposed, to finish, and this year I gave a lot of thought as to why. It was not a race—I knew I could stop at any time—and frankly, I did not have to be running it in the first place. In other words, it was my choice, my pressure, my anxiety. Yet meeting Cyd at the end and piling into the car, dirty, bruised, exhausted, and worn down, I was once again reminded of the profound value of stepping far outside the mundane every now and then. Every so often testing our mettle, we remind ourselves of who we are, what we can do, and, at the very least, that we are not afraid to try. We remind ourselves that we are, in fact, still here.

Last, two random but unexpectedly relevant conversations I'd had in the days leading up to this year's race further sealed the importance of these lessons I've learned—and which I seek to impart to you in this book.

First, I spoke with a friendly guy who coordinates the ambulance that I have on site during the race, graciously donated by our local hospital. He and I were working out the logistics, and I invited him to come down on race day for some food. He had only recently learned about ultramarathons, and after hearing about my race from multiple people in the community, he was struck by how varied the runners were—people seemingly from all walks of life who had come together to toe the line. Of course, it's hard not to acknowledge the diversity of all the people who participate, but it's even more incredible to recognize how similar we all are.

The second conversation was with a couple I'd met at the Stanford Inn just two days before the race. They were checking out the resort as a possible wedding venue, and I was showing them around. Coincidentally—or perhaps fortuitously—they were both trail runners. We chatted about races, ultra-distances, and the trail-running experience specifically. "There is so much time to think," the bride-to-be explained. "Indeed," I thought.

As I wrote throughout this book, trail ultrarunning is truly its own animal. The nature of this singular experience is wonderful but also intimidating and fear-inducing. For most Normal People, it is a vast unknown. But, as I hope each reader who picks this book up believes by now, it *is* something that Normal People can attempt and even conquer. In a truly tangible sense, running in nature and pushing our limits are built into our DNA. Both are part of who we are as a species, and we would all do well to reclaim them both.

Training Tips

I just leave my door and see where my legs take me for the day.

— COURTNEY DAUWALTER, ONE OF THE GREATEST PROFESSIONAL ULTRARUNNERS OF ALL TIME

A Normal Person's first ultramarathon is the hardest to train for because they must navigate the fear of the unknown on top of the training. There isn't even a similar past experience on which to draw from. As such, it makes perfect sense to seek solace in a training plan and to, in a sense, have someone else tell you exactly what to do and when. As we know by now, the hitch is that Normal People live normal lives with jobs, kids, schedules, obligations, and responsibilities. We cannot afford to put significant areas of our normal lives on hold to train. Though this fact does not render training plans useless, it means that approaching them with flexibility and versatility in mind will enable more successful outcomes.

My best advice to all Normal People pursuing ultramarathons is to pay close attention to and manage their stress during training, and not just in relation to the running component. Overall stress—how we are sleeping, our moods, our levels of fatigue when we are not running or training, our abilities to focus at work and in other important areas of our lives—contributes to the success (or lack of success) of a training plan. The bottom line is that any training plan should be used merely as a guideline, rather than a rule. Not only is it okay to take unscheduled days off but it is also advantageous. If on a given day you are just not feeling it, it is better for your long-term goal—not only of finishing the ultramarathon but also of maintaining your overall health—to take a rest day or to do much less than what the training plan might have had in store for you, rather than pushing through it. You can always run less, take a walk, practice some yoga, do some light strength training, or simply do nothing at all and come back swinging the next day.

In your day-to-day life, this means not pushing forward on a workout, such as your training plan's run, if you didn't sleep well the night before or if you just aren't feeling that great in general. It means having the freedom to adjust, adapt, and change your training plan from time to time if your life dictates the need to do so—considering situations like parties, travel, a longer-than-expected workday, and more. Remember, no training plan in a book knows you personally. The plan does not know how well you recover from stress (of any kind), how healthy you eat, how demanding your job is, how long your commute is, how busy your family is, how active your social life is, or how healthy your sleep hygiene is. When choosing a training plan, find one from a reputable source but do the work of making it your own by customizing it to your life and goals as needed.

That said, let's explore some recommendations regarding training for your first ultramarathon, through the lens of continuing with the sport after the first attempt. The goal is to have a positive experience, both physically and mentally, such that you want to do it again and again.

Training for an ultramarathon

Below are my basic training benchmarks. An aspect I love about ultrarunning is that there's no getting around the work that it takes to cross the finish line. So these benchmarks can't be hacked, but that's half of the fun anyways.

Get in the miles

At the end of the day, you could toss out any training plan and spend four to six months steadily building your distances and fitness. For a 50K, I recommend a peak of forty to fifty miles per week, and for a fifty-miler, fifty to sixty miles run overall per week. Keep in mind that these are the peak miles, meaning you might only hit those weekly distances a few of the weeks during your training.

Here is an example of how the weekly mileage might play out, starting with the shorter distances and building over time to the longer ones: running four to eight miles during the week, then running five to twenty miles on the weekends. Of course, this is a large range, but progressively increasing the mileage over time will get you gradually more comfortable with the longer distances. Start with three or four miles on weekdays and five or six miles on one of the weekend days. The longest runs during your entire training need only be just over half of the race distance. For instance, if you are training for a 50K (31.4 miles), your longest run should hover around the eighteen-to-twenty-mile mark. Begin with two days off per week (one weekday, one weekend day), then transition to just one day off per week once you are a couple months into training.

During training, I recommend two taper weeks, weeks with significantly less mileage (four to eight miles total for the week) that give your body and mind a little recovery time. The first taper week should occur about two months prior to race day, and the second should occur the week leading up to the race. The purpose of the prerace taper week is both to prepare your body for race day and to "shake out" the prerace jitters with easy, relaxing runs.

If you were expecting a fancy training chart, here is my anti-chart sell to Normal People. *Not* having a chart to follow and on which to check off each run gives you space to establish a real connection to how you *feel* during training. To run a Normal Person's successful race, it is imperative not only to train but to avoid overtraining. I cannot stress enough how crucial it is to back off the training plan as needed if and when you feel you might be heading into physical or mental overwhelm. There is no denying the comfort of a training plan, but the practice of checking in with yourself every day and adjusting the plan accordingly is invaluable for ultrarunning training and for living an always-in-training life. By maintaining consistent control over the quality and quantity of your training runs, you will be able to manage your stress more effectively, which will in turn ensure both a successful race and postrace recovery. At the end of the day, of course, you must get the miles in. The difference I'm advocating for—over blindly adhering to a training plan—is to get them in while maintaining a strong baseline of health and happiness and effectively managing stress at the same time.

One last note on these miles: you should take them nice and slow. A good gauge for this approach is to ensure you could have a conversation and that you can maintain nasal breathing while running. These relatively easy runs make up the foundation of your fitness and endurance, so keep them as the bulk of your training.

Mix it up

As you now know, running a trail is a very different animal than running on a road. You will inevitably engage more muscle groups on trails, so it is always best to train with this fact in mind. I recommend most of your training to be on actual trails whenever possible, but if this is a challenge (for instance, if you live in a city without easy access to trails), periodically incorporate the following training modifications into your training regimen to mock how the trails will physically challenge you. But keep in mind that the more time you can train on trails, the less you need to be concerned with any of these modifications, as you will be getting them naturally on the trails themselves. I would recommend scattering in these modifications at most one or two times per week on average. If you feel a need to include more, reread the first benchmark.

Strength training

I recommend incorporating functional strength training—exercises that use multiple muscle groups at once—with a specific focus on the adductors and abductors (muscles used for side-to-side movement). It's also important to integrate squats, lunges, and some core work, including both abdominal exercises and back strength exercises. I use the TRX Suspension Trainer and Rip Trainer, but resistance bands are inexpensive and effective as well. Simple bands and hand weights can be used at home and cover the same ground.

Hill repeats

After a warm-up of a mile or two, repeat some uphill runs, running speedily up the hill, then jogging lightly back down, five to eight times followed by a cooldown. Alternatively, you can plan a hilly training run and take the hills with a little more gusto. However, as with trails, finding hills can be a challenge in some cities. Thankfully, stairs can solve this problem. Eric Schranz, host of the *Ultrarunner Podcast*, told me he runs up parking structure ramps to get hill training in his relatively flat city.

Interval runs

After the warm-up miles, significantly increase your pace for one to two minutes, lightly jog to recover for a minute, then repeat five to eight times, followed by a cooldown jog.

Hikes

Some ultramarathon courses include hills so steep that, for Normal People and even some pros, it is more efficient to hike them than to run them. Because hiking necessitates a different stride and gait, spend some training days going on long hikes, leaving the running for another day.

Downhill runs

Toward the end of ultramarathons, running downhill is often more taxing than running uphill. The pounding on the quads can be quite uncomfortable and even debilitating. During training, make sure to get plenty of downhill running in. For trail runs, I recommend occasionally alternating between running up hills and hiking down, then hiking up hills and running down. The overall goal is to engage and develop multiple muscle groups.

Run on tired legs

As we covered in the previous benchmark, your longest run should be around half of your race distance. When I toed the line at the fifty-miler, I had run only thirty-one miles previously, and only once before. Though this may be surprising to some, this approach is completely normal to trail ultrarunning, especially when you're just starting out. Remember that during your training, you will be running substantial distances each week, but the miles are spread out—over five to six days. Race day, on the other hand, occurs at the tail end of a light taper week, which gives your muscles enough time to rest and recover.

Refrain from running the full race distance during training because it just takes too much out of you and isn't part of a proper training regimen. But make no mistake, on that first race day it will be physically and mentally challenging to run longer than you ever have. Thankfully, the energy and excitement of the race and being among other runners will be a huge boost, neither of which you have during training. However, you can prepare for the challenge of running distances on tired legs by scattering in some back-to-back long runs. You need only to take this approach three or four times during your entire training to see the benefits. For example, in lieu of one eighteen- or nineteen-mile run on a given week, run a twelve-miler on Saturday and another twelve-miler on Sunday—or some other version of that type of split, such as a twelve-miler, then a fourteen-miler on another day. Back-to-back runs get you very familiar with running on tired legs and are a great confidence builder. But don't attempt back-to-back long runs until you are deep into your training. A couple or so months in, after you have transitioned to six days a week, might be a good time to attempt your first back-to-back long run.

I remember well my first back-to-back long run. It was over my birthday weekend when I ran a twelve-miler on Saturday, and I was absolutely dreading the twelve-miler that I was set to do the next day, on my actual birthday. I reluctantly got up early Sunday morning and began. While I was definitely feeling the strain of tired muscles for the first five to ten minutes, I settled into a surprisingly enjoyable run. The run was definitely a confidence-building experience, and after I had a great appreciation for what the human body is capable of.

Eat well

One of the most overlooked aspects of training, especially by Normal People, is healthy eating. As noted, many Normal People assume that with the increased training, they can afford to eat whatever, but that isn't the case. In fact, the opposite is true: additional training means additional stress, and to cope with this additional stress, your body needs high-quality nutritional support. It's important to get more calories in to account for the increased energy expenditure, but the quality of those calories matters too. Some coaches and personal trainers focus solely on calories from the macronutrients or "macros," protein, fat, carbohydrates. But this approach is uninformed and, frankly, dangerous. Protein is certainly a vital component to nutrition, but a disproportionally large societal emphasis on protein—an emphasis devoid of a scientific basis and one that fails to account for the fact that most humans consume too much protein—has steered us wrong. Thankfully, it's easy to eat well and get the quantity of calories necessary not only to fuel the body but to fuel it well. Normal People need to consider the quality of calories, as in calories from junk food versus calories from healthy food choices, because we have normal lives to live before and after the race.

As a nutritionist, I have established a specific nutritional approach, largely focused on what does or does not come packaged *with* the calories and macronutrients, instead of placing all the emphasis on the calories themselves. To illustrate this, to provide an accessible way to understand food and what truly determines how healthy a given food is (spoiler alert: it has nothing to do with protein), I think of food as a gift box.

When we receive a gift, the first thing we do is unwrap it and discard the wrapping paper. We do this because the wrapping paper is simply what we use to identify the box we have just been given as a present.

Beyond that, the wrapping paper does not make much difference to us, so we discard it. Why? We want to know what is inside the box because that is where the value of the gift resides. If we open the box and there is not much in there, we will be disappointed, regardless of how nice the wrapping paper was. On the other hand, when we open the box to find something valuable inside, we will think it is a great gift, regardless of the wrapping paper.

Now imagine every food is a gift box covered in wrapping paper. The wrapping paper of food is the calories, the energy, the macronutrients—some form of carbohydrate, fat, or protein, or a combination of these. Some foods have only one form. For example, the wrapping paper of white sugar is all carbohydrate, the wrapping paper of oil is all fat, the wrapping paper of protein powder is all or almost entirely protein. Others have two forms. For example, beef's wrapping paper is usually some protein and mostly fat, with no carbohydrates. Others contain all three. For example, the wrapping paper of spinach is made up of mostly protein and carbohydrate, with a little fat. However, as with an actual gift box, food's wrapping paper is simply how you know it is food, but it does not determine the value or health of the food. In other words, if an object has a form of energy that the human body can convert into usable energy, it is food. But this does not tell us anything about whether that food is healthy. The health, or value, of the food resides inside the "box."

As such, once we "unwrap" the food and take a look at the contents inside, we may find nothing of value, a hugely valuable gift, or something in between. Inside the food gift box, we might find fiber and micronutrients—vitamins, minerals, phytochemicals, antioxidants. The more of these in the box, the healthier the food. Therefore, it is the presence or absence of micronutrients and fiber that determines the health of any given food. Put simply, the wrapping paper tells us whether an object is food or not, but what is inside the box tells us how healthy that food is.

When I teach my classes on nutrition and healthy living, I talk about "light-box foods" and "heavy-box foods." Light-box foods are foods that don't contain much inside the box. Light-box foods will run our bodies, but they won't run them well. If these foods make up the bulk of our diets, we increase the chance of breakdown. Heavy-box foods, on the other hand, will also run our bodies, but they will run them well. When heavy foods make up the bulk of our diets, we will move better and sleep better, achieve better moods, benefit from more robust immune systems, and have healthier microbiomes robust with beneficial gut bacteria. Vitamins, minerals, phytochemicals, antioxidants, and fiber all help the body to function optimally and efficiently and in a comparatively lower-stress state. These are the food ingredients that help our machines run smoothly, while our bodies run on energy in the form of calories.

The lightest-box foods on the planet are refined foods—foods that used to be heavy-box foods until humans threw most of the contents of the box away, leaving an empty or near-empty box. No refined foods can be found in nature. For instance, we will never stumble upon refined white sugar in the wild. Examples of light-box foods are added sugar, all oils, butter, white rice, white flour, and protein powders. These are all extremely light boxes because in creating these refined foods, we've removed almost all, if not all, of the micronutrients that were originally present in the box. For example, we take an olive that contains protein, fat, and carbohydrate for its wrapping paper, and vitamins, minerals, phytochemicals, antioxidants, fiber, and water inside its box, then refine the fat out it and toss out almost everything that was in the box, including all of the fiber. Olive oil is 100 percent fat, as all oils are, and a very light box.

The next heaviest on the spectrum are animal foods. Eggs and flesh have fat and protein but no carbohydrates—one reason those on the dangerous so-called keto diet love them—while dairy has all three macros. Inside the boxes of animal foods, you will find substantially more value and varying amounts of vitamins, minerals, and antioxidants, though no phytochemicals nor fiber. The weight of a given animal-food box depends on how healthy the animal eats: the healthier the animal, the healthier the animal product, which makes wild-animal foods heavier boxes than factory-farmed animal foods.

The next heaviest are whole plants. In order of health, these are as follows: nuts, seeds, whole grains, beans, fruit, then vegetables. All whole plants have all three macronutrients—protein, fat, carbohydrate—and inside the boxes are varying amounts of vitamins, minerals, antioxidants, phytochemicals, and fiber.

Let's review our foods from the lightest to heaviest boxes: refined foods, animal foods, and whole plants. All of these boxes are digestible by the human body; however, the proportion of micronutrients to calories increases as you move along the spectrum. In other words, the value of the gift increases as you move from refined plants all the way up to whole plants—from protein powder to kale.

The one item that may or may not be in the box, and that I have become more and more focused on over the years, is fiber. So much so that focusing on fiber makes basic nutrition even easier to understand and a healthy diet easier to implement. While most people know that fiber helps move things along the digestive track, fiber also regulates the absorption of energy such that the presence of fiber does a fantastic job in preventing wide blood sugar spikes. This is one of the main reasons that people who consume mostly whole plants are not nearly as susceptible to diabetes, even though they consume a high-carbohydrate diet. However, the most important role of fiber in the body is to nourish the healthy gut bacteria in our bodies.

The microbiome—the population of microorganisms in and around our bodies—has garnered more and more attention over the year and rightfully so. Specifically, the good bacteria in our gut play a crucial role in our health and vibrancy. In fact, a healthy gut translates to a more robust immune system, decreased inflammation, improved sleep, improved mood, and better digestion. Maintaining a healthy gut is essential to maintaining a healthy body.

Beyond my light- and heavy-box analogy for food, I teach people this simple truth: food that contains fiber is healthier than food that does not. Fiber resides only in whole plants: nuts, seeds, whole grains, beans, fruits, and vegetables. Not only are whole plants the heaviest-box foods on the spectrum—meaning that they possess the most micronutrients per calorie—but unlike refined plants and animal foods, they all contain fiber. As such, whole plants do the best job of nourishing us *and* the good bacteria inside of us.

Setting aside nostalgia, routine, and ritual (and in many cases, addiction), eating healthy is easy. This means consuming mostly whole plants but not sweating some less healthy foods when time and circumstance dictate: when at parties, out to dinner, out traveling, and even on race day when gels and sports drinks do the trick. In my opinion, the biggest challenge for any Normal Person embarking on training for an ultramarathon is getting enough quality calories. A common mistake people make when eating whole plants is that their portion sizes are not large enough to deliver sufficient calories because whole plants (especially fruits and vegetables) deliver fewer calories than their animal-food and refined-food counterparts when considering their size or volume. For example, a tablespoon of olive oil yields one hundred twenty calories, while the same amount of calories is equal to more than an average entire head of romaine lettuce. The amount of calories from different sources varies widely in terms of size and volume. With this in mind, I advise people to eat much larger portions of vegetables and fruits, then add in whole grains and beans, plus some nuts and seeds. Every human who consumes sufficient calories from whole plants will consume enough protein, fat, and carbohydrates—but more importantly, they'll also consume sufficient micronutrients. If that still surprises you, consider the fact that other animals, like gorillas, consume plenty of protein solely from whole plants. I do recommend most people keep an eye on their consumption of both vitamin B_{12}, which originates in dirt that is washed off our plants, and vitamin D, which our bodies produce with the help of sunlight. Often, it's worth supplementing both of these micronutrients.

All in all, when we exercise more, we must eat more. But Normal People benefit from focusing on the *quality* of their calories—remember to consider how heavy the box is when selecting foods, as much as the quantity of calories you consume. Fuel the body, but fuel it well. Remember, we have more ultramarathons to run and lives to live outside of ultrarunning.

Sleep well

More and more science is emerging on sleep, and there are practical tools to both improve overall sleep and increase deep sleep. Dimming lights at dusk, wearing orange-lensed glasses (blue-light blockers) in the evenings, minimizing or completely discontinuing screen use at night, eating healthy (yes, fiber from whole plants improves sleep), finishing eating about three hours before bedtime, and doing breathwork and meditation all help us to wind down and prepare our bodies and minds for a restorative and restful night. Healthy sleep optimizes training and recovery and should be a key player in any successful ultramarathon training plan. For more resources on beneficial sleep practices, please see the Resources section.

Breathe well

I highly recommend including breathwork as part of your training. As an Oxygen Advantage breathing coach, I am partial to that modality, but there are other great ones out there. I train with almost 100 percent nasal breathing, and I utilize this as a tool during runs as it helps me maintain a *slow* enough and sufficiently low-stress pace and intensity. This, in turn, facilitates and maximizes adaptations in my mind and body. In other words, if I can inhale and exhale through my nose, I am running at a comfortable, sustainable, and beneficial pace. Periodically, switching to mouth breathing will be necessary—for example, during hill repeats and intervals—but, in general, maintaining a pace with which you can calmly inhale and exhale through your nose goes a long way in helping to avoid overtraining.

Resources

Books:

The China Study: The Most Comprehensive Study of Nutrition Ever Conducted and the Starting Implications for Diet, Weight Loss, and Long-Term Health by T. Colin Campbell, PhD and Thomas M. Campbell II

Breath: The New Science of a Lost Art by James Nestor

Born to Run: A Hidden Tribe, Superathletes, and the Greatest Race the World Has Never Seen by Christopher McDougall

Why We Sleep: Unlocking the Power of Sleep and Dreams by Matthew Walker

Eat and Run: My Unlikely Journey to Ultramarathon Greatness by Scott Jurek

Finding Ultra: Rejecting Middle Age, Becoming One of the World's Fittest Men, and Discovering Myself by Rich Roll

Relentless Forward Progress: A Guide to Running Ultramarathons by Bryon Powell

My Work:

Books:

Approaching the Natural: A Health Manifesto

Raising Healthy Parents: Small Steps, Less Stress, and a Thriving Family

Six Truths: Live by These Truths and Be Happy. Don't, and You Won't.

Stress Management and Habit Change Coaching Programs:

smallstepintensive.com (twelve-week private coaching program)

smallsteppers.com (twelve-week online program)

Both programs include nutrition, fitness, and breathwork coaching.

Other Stuff:

sidgarzahillman.com (running and breathwork coaching, videos, and podcast)

Mendocino Coast 50K at www.mendocinoultra.com

youtube.com/sidgarzahillman

What Sid Thinks Podcast (my current podcast)

Approaching the Natural Podcast (my previous podcast)

FAQ

I'm considering trying an ultramarathon for the first time, and there are so many races out there. What makes a good first race?

Try finding a middle-of-the-road race with regard to elevation, terrain, and weather (i.e., not in Death Valley in the middle of summer). But also, and perhaps more importantly, find a race that is beautiful and in an accessible location. Logistics do matter in the context of the stress and anxiety leading up to a race. Consider how easy travel will be to and from the race, how close hotels are to the start, and whether the course is a loop or a point-to-point race. Point-to-point races require having to take a shuttle back to the start, whereas loops mean your car is waiting for you when you finish the race. Personally, I have not enjoyed waiting for a shuttle, nor sitting in a crammed bus, on the way back to the starting line.

Do I need to run a 10K, a half-marathon, and full marathon before attempting a trail ultramarathon?

The short answer is no. This may sound crazy, but recall that trail running is a completely different animal. In other words, road races and trail races are apples and oranges. I have had plenty of runners in my own race for whom this is their first race ever—as in, ne'er a 10K, half-marathon, etc. No matter what, an ultramarathon will require a unique training regimen and will be an experience unlike that of any road race. On the other hand, one can definitely gain confidence from completing a road marathon, but it is not a requirement one must satisfy before attempting an ultra.

There are no training/mileage charts in this book, but I feel better about the idea of having a clear running training chart, especially for a first race. What should I do?

I specifically did not want this book to be a straight-up running guide. My goal was to delve into the philosophy and mindset of ultrarunning, so I intentionally veered away from anything overtly guide-focused. That said, I completely understand the need for this, and thankfully there are a ton of great ultrarunning guidebooks out there. (Please see the Resources section.) However, I still maintain that a Normal Person's success will hinge on our ability to be fluid and versatile in our training. My concern about indiscriminately following a chart is that it prevents us from being in tune with ourselves. If we have a "versatile" mindset, charts can work well *and* if we prioritize checking in with ourselves before each training run: How did I sleep? How am I feeling? How fatigued am I? How busy is my workday coming up? Am I in pain?

Forging ahead with what the chart says without asking these questions can easily lead to overtraining and possibly injury. Always remember: you are in charge of your training, not the other way around.

Do I need to hire a coach?

I had a great experience working with a coach, but for me the benefit was much more about what I learned regarding versatility and adaptability. I did not have a coach during the entirety of my training, just to point me in the right direction. Having a coach can be a great support and a confidence builder, and with that accountability in place, the training experience can be less stressful, but hiring a coach is absolutely not necessary.

Training with friends can yield some of the same benefits in terms of accountability and fun.

I live in a city, and with my work schedule, I can only get time on a treadmill. Is it possible to still finish a trail ultra?

Absolutely, but you'll still need the miles, and strength training is essential. Trails tax multiple muscle groups in a way that treadmills cannot, so adding in full-body training (with lunges, squats, side-to-side band workouts, etc.) will go a long way toward preparing you. Last, mix up the treadmill workouts from time to time. For instance, once or twice per week, work with varying inclines and declines (if your treadmill is equipped for declines) and varying speeds. The other days, take it nice and easy, focusing on proper running form while going slowly enough to facilitate full nasal breathing.

I'm super busy, and training for an ultra seems like it'd be way too much for me to take on.

There is no getting around the fact that training for an ultra will require additional time and energy. As with any relatively short-term challenge (diets included), training requires some rearranging of schedules, additional help from friends and family, etc. However, I have successfully trained for multiple races with a family, a full-time job (or even more than one), and more obligations. The shifts, while necessary, do not have to be massive. Getting up a littler earlier goes a long way in allowing training to occur without major upset to your regular life. As a running coach, I find that most people are overtraining and can get away with far less mental and physical strain during training. As a result, I laid out some basic training and mileage guidelines, and I urge you to revisit them.

Yes, you will be a little more tired than usual (both from a little less sleep and from more exercise), but this is the nature of putting yourself out there—of testing your mettle. When you cross the finish line, you will know exactly why you decided to attempt this in the first place.

Are there any inherent physical or mental attributes that make someone more successful at ultrarunning?

Success for a Normal Person ultrarunner means training intelligently, managing stress effectively, toeing the line, and doing our best to finish. In this way, there is no need for special talent or any inherent physical or mental attributes, except perhaps a desire to step outside of what you know and are comfortable with. I have seen a diverse range of shapes, sizes, and ages crossing my finish line. Approaching ultrarunning in the way I have advocated for in this book will significantly increase your chances of having a life-changing and profoundly positive experience.

Do you eat during the race? If so, what?

You will definitely need to eat during any ultramarathon—the sheer distance and time you're on the trails require calories well beyond what you eat before the starting gun fires. What ultrarunners eat, however, varies widely. Some stick to gels and sports drinks, others try potatoes, cookies, peanut butter and jelly sandwiches, fruit—and the list goes on! One thing to keep in mind is that often the food you plan on consuming during a race—gels, for example—starts to lose its appeal after many hours, so do not be afraid to go for something you crave as you get closer to the finish. I remember arriving at an aid station at about mile twenty-six of a 50K and having an intense craving for Coca-Cola! I drank some, and it was to this day one of the best things ever!

Experiment with different foods during training and find out what you like and don't like, what upsets your stomach or not, etc. It is important to understand that stress weakens digestion, which is a big reason that gels and sports drinks are so effective on race day as they are super easy to digest.

How do you handle bathroom breaks?

During an ultramarathon, there's a very good chance that nature will be your bathroom. Throw a little toilet paper in your pocket, and if necessary, peel off the trail and take care of business. Some races have porta potties at points along the course— at my race, on the other hand, runners will not see one until about mile twenty-four. There is a silver lining: nobody cares. Remember, we're all in this together, and it is just a thing wild animals do in nature. On race day, on trails, and in the midst of fatigue, think of yourself as a wild animal. It's kind of liberating, actually (and on some level, true).

What are the major risks of running an ultramarathon?

If you train well, effectively manage your stress and life prior to race day, shoot for a Normal Person's success (i.e., not looking at your watch), and maintain awareness and attention, you will most likely avoid major risk. You might take a fall, stub a toe, cramp, throw up if and when you overconsume a beverage or food, experience nausea, etc., but creating an environment of wild attention means actually being able to listen to your body. You may need to drop out of a particular race because not doing so would be risking too much. This is not only okay but it's the right thing to do. If you truly cannot go on, here is what you do: go back to the drawing board, retool your training, and try again.

Acknowledgments

A big, big thank you . . .

To the entire Blue Star Press team, with special thanks to:

Brenna Licalzi for taking a chance on this book (a philosophy of ultrarunning?!?).

Lindsay Wilkes-Edrington for excellent guidance, care, attention, and a hyphenated last name.

Avalon Radys for being an incredible editor and advisor.

Hanna Richards for fine-tuning and tightening (and for an otherworldly eye for detail!).

To Skip Brand for writing the foreword and joining me every year for our pre-race day 50K course run and marking tradition. The Mendocino Coast 50K could not happen without you and your team at Healdsburg Running Company.

To Cyd Ross and Brie Robertson—my good friends and training partners—for repeatedly getting me out on the trails.

And finally to my family: Lisa, Luna, Rónán, and Rinah for your love and support.

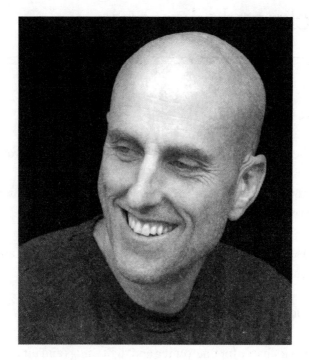

Author Bio

Sid Garza-Hillman is the author of published works, *Approaching the Natural: A Health Manifesto*; *Raising Healthy Parents: Small Steps, Less Stress, and a Thriving Family*; and *Six Truths: Live by These Truths and Be Happy. Don't, and You Won't.* He is a public speaker, podcaster, certified nutritionist and running coach, and an Oxygen Advantage® breathing instructor. He is the Stanford Inn & Resort's wellness programs director, founder of Small Steppers, and race director of the Mendocino Coast 50K trail ultramarathon.